Dear Da

KALEIDOSCOPE

Our good fried Alan
thought you might
be intresked in
radeig my first published
book — I hope you
enjoy'd!

Many thanks for your
intres

Barbara Evans

KALEIDOSCOPE

Barbara Erasmus

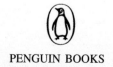

PENGUIN BOOKS

PENGUIN BOOKS

Published by the Penguin Group
80 Strand, London WC2R 0RL, England
Penguin Putnam Inc, 375 Hudson Street, New York, New York 10014, USA
Penguin Books Australia Ltd, 250 Camberwell Road, Camberwell,
Victoria 3124, Australia
Penguin Books Canada Ltd, 10 Alcorn Avenue, Toronto, Ontario,
Canada M4V 3B2
Penguin Group (NZ), Cnr Airborne and Rosedale Roads, Albany,
Auckland 1310, New Zealand
Penguin Books India (P) Ltd, 11 Community Centre, Panchsheel Park,
New Delhi – 110 017, India
Penguin Books (South Africa) (Pty) Ltd, 24 Sturdee Avenue, Rosebank,
Johannesburg 2196, South Africa

Penguin Books (South Africa) (Pty) Ltd, Registered Offices:
24 Sturdee Avenue, Rosebank, Johannesburg 2196, South Africa

First published by Penguin Books (South Africa) (Pty) Ltd 2004

Copyright © Barbara Erasmus 2004

All rights reserved
The moral right of the author has been asserted

ISBN 0 143 02448 5

Typeset by CJH Design in 10.5/13 pt
Cover design: Flame Design, Cape Town
Printed and bound by Interpak Books, Pietermaritzburg

Except in the United States of America, this book is sold subject to the
condition that it shall not, by way of trade or otherwise, be lent, resold, hired
out or otherwise circulated without the publisher's prior consent in any form
of binding or cover other than that in which it is published and without a
similar condition including this condition being imposed on the subsequent
purchaser.

For Michael, Nics and Luc

KALEIDOSCOPE

'Tube through which are seen symmetrical figures,
produced by reflections of pieces of coloured glass etc.,
and varied by rotation of the tube; (fig.) constantly
changing group of bright or interesting objects'.
The Concise Oxford Dictionary

In Broken Images

He is quick, thinking in clear images;
I am slow, thinking in broken images.

He becomes dull, trusting to his clear images;
I become sharp, mistrusting my broken images.

Trusting his images, he assumes their relevance;
Mistrusting my images, I question their relevance.

Assuming their relevance, he assumes the fact;
Questioning their relevance, I question the fact.

When the fact fails him, he questions his senses;
When the fact fails me, I approve my senses.

He continues, quick and dull in his clear images;
I continue, slow and sharp in my broken images.

He is in a new confusion of his understanding;
I am in a new understanding of my confusion.

Robert Graves

Prologue

As a child, I won a kaleidoscope at the beach kiosk. The pavement felt warm against my bare, sandy feet as I stood, mesmerised by interlocking shapes and colours, boundaries which shifted at my touch. I remember Kate's impatient fingers on my arm, her dancing feet.

'Come on Claire! You're causing a traffic jam!'

Kate was never still. Her name was really Katherine. You can do a lot with a word like Katherine. My mother used to tuck her into bed, love-names tripping off her tongue. Katie. Kit-cat. Katherine-wheel. I listened as I lay next door, cool between my solitary sheets. I didn't like tickling. No giggling in my room. Claire's not as malleable a name as Katherine. It's a single syllable. You can't make it shorter. Or longer. It's not playful. I've never heard a song about a girl called Claire.

I was overshadowed – even by her name.

Kate's segment in a kaleidoscope would be red. It's a loud colour. For energy. For warmth. Chaos and disruption. She'd be a hexagon, at the very least. Multi-sided, many-angled. A red hexagon – making a major impact, dominating the final pattern. I'm more a triangle, I think. Sharp edged and dyed an icy, keep-your-distance blue. Not equilateral. Long sides for work and application. Short on relationships. Like Tony – no colour at all for him. Sepia perhaps – like a faded movie, a background filler. No one notices he's in the picture. Amy's different. She'd be a circle – you can't get inside a circle. It's exclusive – no angles or joints where seepage could occur. Her colours can't be classified.

My mind's selective when it recalls my early childhood. Most of it's gone forever. But I remember my kaleidoscope with its interlocking fragments and shifting perspectives.

Perhaps it was a glimpse of the future.

Interlocking fragments . . .

Claire : Ice-blue. Triangular.

I've always had a phenomenal memory – for certain things. I'm not much good at general knowledge. I can't lay claim to an encyclopaedic grasp of art or music. Lists are my speciality – rows of unrelated items. I've always liked lists. The Oxford Dictionary is my bible. I'm very familiar with the Oxford – I relate more to a dictionary than to a novel.

I remember lists verbatim.

I learned to keep this talent hidden when I saw how it unnerved my mother. I've a clear recollection of an early incident at Pick 'n Pay. I was about seven years old – Kate must have been five. My mother was having a dinner party. Perhaps that's why it stands out in my memory – my parents seldom entertained. Our dining room table was littered with cookery books as my mother planned her menu. Nothing too risky, she told me. Fillet with wine and mushrooms, followed by a baked cheesecake – my grandmother's recipe never failed. I was sitting beside her as she wrote down the ingredients she needed. 1 kilogram fillet. 2 cloves garlic. 5 millilitres mustard. 200 milligrams olive oil. 6 sprigs of thyme. 200 grams mushrooms. And so on . . .

Kate was whining by the time we got to Pick 'n Pay. My mother rashly bribed Kate with a trolley of her own. She might as well have handed over a loaded machine gun. Kate tore off down the aisle as if it was a Grand Prix circuit, stretching up on tiptoe for tempting tins and packets – she's always been drawn to anything out of reach. My mother and I scrambled in her wake, anticipating chaos. Kate and a supermarket were not a winning combination. My mother was already stressed about the dinner party. She ran her fingers through her hair as she rummaged in her handbag with a feverish expression.

'I don't know why I ever write a list,' she told me. 'I can never find it when I get here.'

'1 kilogram fillet,' I said helpfully. '2 cloves garlic. 5 millilitres mustard . . .'

She'd spoken out loud when she wrote down her list of ingredients. I could remember every single item. In the right order. Order is important to me. I worked my way through both the main course and the cheesecake. I thought my mother would be pleased when she heard my recitation. She said she was pleased. She said I was a clever girl. But she looked bemused.

I heard her talking to Ruth on the phone that evening.

3

Ruth was her sister. They were as close as Kate and I were distant. She didn't see me standing in the passage. She had her back to me. She thought I was in bed.

'Claire's so strange,' she said. 'David says I'm making an issue out of nothing. He says he's more worried about Kate. She's like a demolition squad. But at least Kate's childish. Claire sometimes gives me the creeps. It's not normal. She's only seven years old, for God's sake. She can't even read. She shouldn't be memorising grocery lists. She's obsessive. Her china animals – they're always in exactly the same place on her shelf. She doesn't play with them. She just arranges them in rows. Over and over again. I dusted the shelf last week and Claire absolutely freaked out when she got home from school. Nothing was broken or missing. They just weren't in the same order. She cried and stamped her feet – she was absolutely distraught. In a way, I was glad to see her showing some emotion for a change.'

She paused to listen to Ruth's reaction. Then she continued. 'You're right. I know she's only little. But it does worry me. I found the bloody list when I got home. She didn't leave out a single thing. And it wasn't muddled. She said it in the order I'd written it. I feel as if I've given birth to a wizard. And a demolition squad. I'm not a very success-ful breeder,' she laughed ruefully. 'I don't know how parents survive their children's childhood.'

I remember that conversation as accurately as the groceries that caused it.

Claire's so strange.

She's obsessive.

It's not normal.

She gives me the creeps.

I've never forgotten it. Lists are my speciality.

✳

Career choice defines a person. It creates an automatic expectation. You learn the art of stereotype as early as the classroom. You expect the art teacher to pitch up with braided hair and orange socks. Maths is pearls and a cashmere sweater. A guy in advertising stands out in a line-up of banker suspects. No one takes housewives seriously. Because they don't get paid for what they do, it's not rated as a real job. Without career definition, you're irrelevant.

Some of these stereotypes are statistically valid. You can trust my opinion here – statistics are my currency. I'm an actuary. Kate's an actor. Just four letters separate my career from hers but semantically, the terms are light years apart – fundamentally different, despite their common core. A single word gives a precis of all that we are. You know everything about us now.

I'm an archetypal mathematician – rigorously precise. It's ironic that I deal with risk when I never take one. Except for Amy – I took a gamble with her. I knew the odds were stacked against me. The concept of probability is one of the fundamental notions of modern science. In my profession, we use the experience of the past to measure the chances of the future. I compute the probabilities of the contingencies of life. Birth. Death. Marriage. Sickness. Loss. They're not emotive terms to me. They're just statistics.

Kate's different – but only in a way. Love and loss are her source material too. I add them up. She acts them out. Maybe we have more in common than we think. We share the same gene pool, after all. Amy showed us that. My poor parents – it must be exhausting for them to contemplate their extension of the family tree. We're certainly diverse. Kate spells trouble. I'm just strange.

My parents don't understand me. No one does. I sound like the proverbial teenager – an embryo adult, groping towards the future, uncertain of the direction I should choose. But I'm not a teenager any longer and I can understand my parents' reservations. I've no complaints about my childhood. My parents did nothing to suggest that Kate was the favourite – I don't think she was. It's more a question of semantics. Love and adore could be synonyms but somehow the nuance is completely different. Love seems more remote. It's listed in the Oxford as a noun as well as a verb. Perhaps that's what makes the difference – it's a concept more than an action. Like pride. My parents are certainly proud of us – we're both achievers, in our different ways. I know they love me and they love Amy too.

But they adore Kate. No one will ever adore Amy or me. It's too tumbled a word for us. Kate's the only one who inspires adoration in our family.

She was always in trouble as a girl. Her room was a health risk – piles of discarded clothes or abandoned sandwiches. School reports despaired of progress. She was either on the phone or in detention. Her music was loud and never-ending. Boyfriends and girlfriends. Shrieks of laughter. Slamming doors and temper tantrums. Kate's life was littered with human contact.

I was on a different planet. The solar system I evolved in was orderly. My planets moved in a regular orbit. No comets collided in my universe. I was the only person living there and it suited me. I don't like clutter. I don't even like conversation. I should be a convicted felon – I'd thrive in solitary confinement, waiting for the noose.

I don't know why. It's not because I'm shy or inarticulate. I'm a competent public speaker. I don't use notes because I never forget what I've prepared. My speeches are well researched with flawless punctuation but they'll never whip a crowd into a frenzy. I won't lead a revolution because I can't ad-lib. Spontaneity is not my forte.

That's why I'm mesmerised by Kate on stage. She's like a chameleon. She slips into whatever role she's playing and makes it seem authentic. She isn't my wayward sister then. She's Eliza with a grimy face and cockney accent. Ophelia, imploding with madness. Harold Pinter's Ruth – mysterious, ambiguous. You can hear the silence as she spins her magic web. She's the only reason I go to the theatre. I don't get much out of watching a performance. I'm never moved to tears and I never rock with laughter – I was dealt a smaller spectrum of emotions than Kate. She and Michael veer from hurling plates to passionate reconciliation. I find them exhausting.

But I'm not jealous when I watch Kate take her curtain calls. I've no desire to be on stage. I've never given a public performance on the piano, even though I passed Grade 8 with flying colours. My mother believed in equal opportunity. When Kate started her drama lessons, I was sent off to music. Separate but equal was part of the family ethos. I made quick progress because I have perfect pitch. I can relate each note I hear to its predecessor. And its successor. Higher or lower – it makes no difference to me. I can identify a single isolated note correctly. But I'll never play like Kate acts because the music's only in my ears. It's not in my heart or in my soul. I don't think I was fitted with a soul – the notes are lodged only in my memory. I remember what my piano teacher said to me one day. I was about fourteen at the time and I'd already passed Grade 6.

'Can't you feel the music Claire?' she wailed. 'You're so wooden. You learn everything so quickly. Technically, you're perfect but I'd welcome a few mistakes in exchange for some emotion. I know you can read the notes but I want to hear what they make you feel when you put them all together . . .'

I didn't understand what she meant. Playing the piano didn't make me feel happy or sad. It was a task I carried out because my parents paid for the lessons. I wasn't good at giving names to feelings.

The only one I recognised was the feeling that I was a misfit.

I was very familiar with that.

＊

I'm a slut.

Semantically, it's an interesting word. Only four letters – the mandatory length in English for anything with unsavoury connotations. It sounds more glamorous if you lengthen it. La slutte sounds almost flirtatious – provocative and sensual. Perhaps it's cultural. A French slutte sounds like a coquette, tousled and pouting. The Oxford dismisses the English slut as slovenly and disgusting – a slattern or a hussy.

I'm not your average slut. Those are probably the last words anyone would choose to describe me. I'd be typecast as the vestal virgin in a play. Kate, with her long record of fidelity, looks far more the part than I do. Men are always surprised at how easily they get me into bed. Despite the rumours. No one really believes them. I look untouchable. I seem to belong on a pedestal. I know they talk about me but it sounds like gossip. Each thinks he's the only one who's really done it.

I lost count of the men I slept with before Tony.

I blame Kate. I often use her as a scapegoat. I was overshadowed by my little sister. She was barely in her teens when the boys started phoning. She was only fifteen when she met Michael. I couldn't stay at home browsing through the Oxford while they went off to movies holding hands. It wasn't fair. Kate's always been the ugly sister. I'm the beautiful one. That sounds arrogant but it's true. Beauty's not something you achieve – it's a chance arrangement of features, a fortuitous combination of eyes and skin and cheekbones. I can see I'm beautiful because I have a mirror. It's like maths – you must be good at maths if you get the answers right. Some conclusions are inescapable. Like friends. I knew I had no friends because no one phoned me.

Sex was easier for me than conversation.

I sound like some kind of nymphomaniac but nothing could be further from the truth. The Oxford describes nymphomania as morbid and uncontrolled sexual desire in women. It's even less applicable to me than slut. Control is a key ingredient in my personality – or lack of personality . . .

That's why I hate sex.

It's so uncontrolled. They're always urgent. Heavy

9

breathing. Fumbling. Hair in my face. It feels like an invasion. I was obviously born four billion years too late. The first living cells on earth existed without males. They reproduced by dividing and passing all their genes to their daughters. And I read an article about some small aquatic creatures – bdelloid ratifers – who've continued to evolve for eighty million years without males or sex. They reject sex completely. I've a lot in common with the ratifer.

This attitude is an anachronism in the new millennium. I'm a relic from the days of Queen Victoria. Close your eyes and think of England is my sexual credo. Kate's been in several plays dealing with sexual issues. She had the lead in Arthur Miller's *Broken Glass* when it premiered in Cape Town at Theatre on the Bay. It's about dysfunctional sexual relationships – perhaps that's why I paid attention. I always cut out her reviews – I keep a scrapbook. I've never showed it to anyone but I browse through it sometimes if I've got an hour to spare. Because the play was new, the reviewer discussed the content before going on to rave about Kate's vulnerability, her resilience.

'Miller's point is that the warmth of healthy sexuality is a bond between people that goes beyond personal love or sex. Allow it to freeze and you'll be an outcast from your self and there is no greater loneliness.'

I've no idea what he's talking about.

I don't exhibit any signs of healthy sexuality. I try to cut down on foreplay. Get it over quickly. Kissing is taboo. That wasn't my idea – I got it from Julia Roberts when she was a hooker in *Pretty Woman*. It made sense to me when she said it. The mouth's the most personal orifice, when you think about it. It's where words come out – the route to your thoughts. I know the vagina's linked to the womb but I don't like anything associated with babies. The vagina doesn't lead to anything significant to me. It doesn't matter who goes in there — so long as they don't stay long.

It sometimes seemed like sex would never end. I used to sneak a glance at my watch.

I could write a Masters thesis on the art of faking orgasm.

✳

The Oxford defines orgasm as the climax of sexual excitement. It meant as little to me as an astronaut describing weightless conditions in a spacecraft. Again, it was Kate who made me curious. I'm not suggesting we had an intimate fireside conversation. Kate and I were more likely to become astronauts than to exchange intimacies by the fire. The concept of orgasm surfaced with *The Vagina Monologues*.

It was one of Kate's most stellar performances. A sold-out season at the Downstairs Theatre at Wits. A triumph at the Baxter. I have the reviews pasted in my scrapbook.

'You can't afford to miss the South African version of Eve Ensler's celebrated play,' it started. *'Kate Templeton is glorious — open, hilarious and uninhibited in her handling of what is an undercover topic for conservative South African audiences. It's not a salacious show, despite the contentious title. She slips effortlessly into the different persona of her monologues — the mood is funny, uplifting and moving as the content shifts from one angle to the next. Templeton shows her class in this production. She could hold her own on Broadway.'*

I had to go, despite my reservations.

We were at lunch at my parents' house when the topic first came up. Kate had seen Eve Ensler live in Chicago. She was brimming with feminist enthusiasm on her return. Kate's always keen on causes. 'It's brilliant!' she raved, stabbing the air with her fork to punctuate her point. 'It only lasts about ninety minutes and she goes from pubic hair to Pap smears and orgasmic moans.' It sounded absolutely ghastly. I could see Tony concentrating on his food. Lunch time conversation in his home focused largely on the weather and the price of groceries.

'It won the Obie Award,' she continued. 'It's a global phenomenon. Glenn Close did it in New York and she had two and a half thousand people chanting "cunt" in unison!' Tony's focus on his pumpkin became more marked than ever. 'I'm inspired by the whole V-Day movement,' she enthused.

'What's V-Day?' asked my father, looking as blank as you'd expect from someone of his generation.

'It's a grass roots movement to stop violence against women. There's a piece in the play about a gang rape in Bosnia. It's appalling. There's another piece about family rape. It sounds like a Sunday tabloid in South Africa. At the end of the show, Ensler came on stage and asked everyone who was or knew a victim of violence against women to stand. Half the audience stood up. I bet the whole bloody audience would stand up if I did it here. I've got to find a sponsor.'

Predictably, she went out and found one. Violence against women is a huge issue in South Africa – and Kate makes an armoured tank look ineffectual when she's in commitment mode. The show was billed as *POWA Power* – People

Opposed to Women Abuse was the sponsor. It got front-page coverage and became an in-vogue outing for city socialites.

I've never missed one of Kate's shows. Right from her school days. Tony usually comes too. Nobody who saw us in our sober suits would guess that we're connected to all that energy on stage. But Tony didn't want to go to this one. He said he had to work but I know he couldn't bring himself to watch a play with vagina in the title. Kate has a tendency to star in shows with contentious titles. Tony didn't come to see her in *Shopping and Fucking* either. I'm glad I went to that – even though I think it's a distressing play. Sex can be so desolate. I wonder what Kate thought about it. I'd never discuss a play with her – my literary opinions are tentative and she's always so passionate. A discussion with Kate sometimes feels like encountering a tidal wave. Silence is safer.

That's why Tony is a good theatre companion. He neither demands nor gives an opinion. But he avoids alternative theatre. I think he's anxious that someone from work might see him. The chances of anyone from Irving Life going to a play with either fucking or vagina in the title are statistically zero but Tony doesn't take any chances. He's obviously decided the risk factor's untenable. I also felt embarrassed. I'd never heard the word vagina outside a biology classroom. As Ensler says in the play, it sounds a bit like a disease.

I booked my solitary ticket on the net. I couldn't bring myself to ask the girl at Computicket face to face. It would have felt like booking for a porn show.

I slipped into the back of the crowded theatre just before

they dimmed the lights. The audience seemed predominantly women. All shapes and sizes and ethnic groups. All talking. Expectant. They fell silent when the spotlight picked out Kate on stage. There was no set. Just a few drapes tossed carelessly across a frame behind her. Swathes of velvet. Pink. Purple. Red. She looked striking against them with her cloud of hair. She wore a long, body-hugging dress, barefoot and motionless behind the mike. She held a sheaf of cards in her hands. Her voice sounded uncharacteristically flat and deadpan when she started.

'I *bet you're worried* . . .' she said. I braced myself as she worked her way through vaginal terminology I'd never heard before. Pussy-cat. Fannybro. Cootchy snortch. She became Jewish. An English aristocrat. A sex worker on the streets of New York City. A lesbian. She made me squirm. She made me listen. She made me wonder about secret places where I'd never been.

I was mesmerised by what I heard. I became aware that it was over. People around me were applauding. Standing up. Calling for more. I slipped out quietly into the silence, the applause getting fainter as I made my way to the corner into which I'd slid my car.

'How was it?' Tony asked when I unlocked the door.

'You wouldn't have liked it,' I told him. A major understatement. Tony would have been even more uncomfortable than I was. He and I would have been the only ones not laughing. I'm glad I went on my own. Tony might have distracted me.

I thought about what Kate had said as I lay under my duvet beside Tony later that night. Tony and I had separate beds but we pushed them together to mislead his mother.

We would have chosen separate rooms if it weren't for her. Tony's mother had clear views on everything. A double bed was part of the marriage ethos in her eyes. She was equally committed to regular meals and normal office hours. Success for her was measured in financial terms. She dismissed Kate and Michael because of their twilight hours, their spasmodic employment. We were amazed at how she came to terms with Amy. Sometimes the most predictable people prove the most surprising.

I didn't forget what Kate said about orgasm. I've explored my body since that evening. Tentative fingers. Cautious. Light brush-stroke touches, waking sleeping nerve ends. Breath catching. Growing urgent . . .

Tendrils of pleasure snaking down my limbs.

And then it's over. It only lasts a moment – it doesn't seem enough to topple kings.

But you can't underplay the potency of sex as a motivational factor. History's full of dangerous liaisons – people risk everything for sex. Colour, class or gender – it doesn't seem to matter how high the stakes.

There was a total eclipse of the sun last year and one of the reports said its effects were on a par with sexual climax. Spectators say they never forget it. They want to repeat it. Some disciples follow eclipses all over the world, eager to relive those minutes – but only a total eclipse has that effect, it seems. Even ninety-nine per cent isn't comparable. It must be the same with sex. My involvement in a sexual encounter was never one hundred per cent. It seldom reached even double figures. Sex must have extra dimensions when your emotions are involved. It's like playing the piano, I suppose. You need more than technique to make it memorable.

I knew I'd interrupted when I arrived at Kate's that day — I'd come to drop off Amy. There was a long pause before Michael opened the door. He was wearing only sleeping shorts — bare-chested with his hair in peaks. Kate's eyes were lidded when she joined us in the lounge. She ruffled Amy's hair — but merely as a reflex. Her thoughts were elsewhere. She ran a finger along Michael's arm. Their smile excluded me and Amy.

But I don't wonder what I've missed. I've got used to having Tony beside me — not close enough to invade my boundaries but I like to hear him breathing. Or turning over. It pleases me to know I'm part of a pair. And now there's Amy to talk about so it's even better. I look forward to the early morning or the time before we fall asleep.

The priest said for better or worse and it's proved to be for better in the end. For everyone concerned.

None of the statistics predicted such an outcome.

*

Every life is landmarked by pinnacle events — critical moments that determine a pattern for the future. The International AFIR Colloquium in Tokyo mapped out a route for me and Tony.

I hardly knew him before we set out on our eastern assignment. No one did — even though he was the senior investment consultant at Irving Life. He had a hugely influential job, defining company strategy within appropriate risk margins. His financial acumen was a legend at Irving's. His recommendations made a major impact on the fortunes of shareholders, on the futures of millions of pension-fund members. But no one really knew anything about Tony. He was a colourless man in a nondescript suit, plugged into his computer – keying in statistics, working out the answers. Sending them by email. The Internet is paradise for someone as lacking in people skills as Tony. He can send out statements to his shareholders and field all their queries without a single word to another human being.

Not that conversation was a problem for us on our flight to Tokyo. We didn't even notice that we'd passed through several time zones. We were immersed in my presentation. Irving Life had won the government commission to devise an actuarial model for assessing the impact of AIDS on the South African economy. It was a major coup and I'd devoted the year to the project. I was going to present my predictions on the international stage at the conference. What I said could affect investment on a national level – both the government and Irving Life had a lot riding on this presentation. It had to be perfect.

Tony was an ideal mentor. He's even more attentive to detail than I am. We'd been through every aspect of my model before we left but we did it all again. We wanted to be sure we'd anticipated every potential query. We're focused people so our attention didn't wander. No presentation at the conference was more thoroughly prepared or methodically presented. It gave me my only insight into the adrenaline Kate must feel when the applause washes round her on stage. I'd never been in the limelight before. I'd walked across the stage at school to get the maths prize but no one really paid attention. They were all eager for prizegiving to end so they could go home for the holidays.

They clapped far more when Kate got the drama award. Everyone knew her because they'd all seen the play. No one knew who I was. A maths fundi has no prestige at high school.

But I was the one in the spotlight in Tokyo that day. Not that actuaries are given to wild applause – their clapping was fairly muted but I was aware of respect as I made my way back to my seat. Tony smiled thinly and nodded. I can recognise an accolade when I see one. He was impressed.

I got to know him better during the time we spent in Tokyo. We were the only delegates from South Africa. Neither of us is gregarious so we stuck together. It wasn't a conscious decision. It happened more by default. A familiar face is an anchor in Tokyo – it's the most foreign city I've ever visited.

My first impressions were surprisingly rural as our plane dipped over a network of paddy fields, green with food for a populous nation. I became aware of Tony's anxiety almost as soon as we disembarked at Narita. It's a huge, immaculate airport and the queues move with legendary Japanese efficiency. Tony looked ill at ease under the foreign signposts.

'Where should we go?' he asked me.

He sounded hesitant. It was the first question he'd asked me – he'd specialised in telling me the answers on the plane. He followed me to the sky-train – sleek and litter-free, departing exactly on schedule. I studied Tony's understated profile as it sped silently towards the never-ending sprawl of urban Tokyo. He ignored me completely.

The week I spent with him in Japan was bewildering. It felt like travelling with a downbeat version of Jekyll and

Hyde. He was like a chameleon. The Oxford defines a chameleon as a small prehensile-tailed lizard with the power to change colour according to its surroundings. A variable or inconsistent person. That describes Tony perfectly.

In the aeroplane, discussing my presentation, he was entirely familiar – intelligent, pedantic, absorbed. He was like that at the conference too. He didn't fidget when listening to the other speakers – and actuaries and orators are diametrically opposed. Actuaries don't keep you glued to your seat, eager for the next instalment. My mind wandered sometimes but Tony never lost focus – I could tell from the round-table discussions which followed each presentation. He wasn't meek and mild in the boardroom. His comments were pertinent and incisive. The delegates sat up and paid attention when he made a contribution.

He was entirely different when he stepped into the streets of Tokyo. He seemed to regress by several decades. I felt as if I was escorting a schoolboy. The prehensile aspect of the chameleon definition certainly applied to Tony when he was in unfamiliar territory. He attached himself to me like a limpet. He also seemed dependent on his cellphone. It rang often and the conversations didn't sound like business. Someone in South Africa would be facing a substantial bill on our return. The calls must come from there, I reasoned. No one in Japan speaks English.

I found Tokyo an appropriate city for Jekyll and Hyde. It's a juxtaposition of opposites – functional, western architecture, side by side with ancient shrines. Ugly concrete buildings, interspersed with magnificent, structured gardens, dating back to distant eras. You have to change gears all the time as you explore. Tony liked traditional Japan. He's not a modern man, in spite of his cyberspace connections. He was daunted by the neon hieroglyphics. Noisy streets jammed with cars and pedestrians. I could see beads of sweat on his forehead as we stood at the Shibuya crossing, waiting for the lights to change. I had to take his arm and lead him forward into the relentless human wave that spilled from the interlocking streets. He didn't seem to notice the famed Shibuya girls with their garish orange hair, white painted faces. Outrageous punk was wasted on Tony.

He perspired even more at dinner when our waitress handed us the incomprehensible menu. You can hazard a guess in Europe but it's a lost cause in Japan. Despite plastic replicas of the food featured in all restaurant windows, I had no idea what to expect when I placed our order. 'I'll have the same as you,' was Tony's only contribution to the crisis. Kate and Michael would have loved eating in Japan. Conveyor belts of sushi. *Sansai-ryori* – fiddlehead ferns, wild fungi and sweetfish. Unfamiliar tastes. We ordered *kamameshi* – a rice casserole with vegetables and chicken. Everyone shouts in Japan. The waiters. The cooks. The Japanese diners. It was overwhelming.

The next night we had hamburgers at McDonald's. We felt safer.

Safety was a big issue for Tony, I realised, as the days grew into a week. A tour had been arranged for all the delegates and I saw Tony relax as he settled back in the seat of the luxury bus, secure in the knowledge that the tour guide would be making all the decisions. Organised tours appeared to be the brand of travel he was used to.

Tony's credo was specialisation. The Oxford defines a speciality as a pursuit to which a person gives special attention. Biologically, to specialise implies adapting to a particular purpose. That's how Tony saw life. He was a specialist in actuarial science. That's what he was good at so that was what he did. It was the only thing he did. Other specialists could tell him where to go and what to eat. These weren't choices he'd had to make himself.

I hadn't met his lifeskills mentor at that stage.

But I felt oddly at ease with Tony. We were both misfits. It felt comfortable to be with someone whose conversational expectations seemed even lower than my own. Our Kyoto guide was offhand about the charms of Philosopher's Pathway. 'It's the wrong season,' she explained. 'It's magnificent in spring when the cherry blossom is massed and fragrant. It looks like a Persian carpet in autumn, rich in shades of red and brown and gold. But no one goes in summer. It's not worth it.'

But Tony and I liked it. We slipped away from the crowded temple and strolled along the quiet bank, emphatically green and lush with cherry trees. We didn't miss the slow-moving throng of tourists. We sipped iced-tea from tall glasses in an empty pavement café. It was pleasant – that's defined as agreeable to mind, feelings and senses.

The Oxford always says precisely what I mean.

Afterwards, the tour bus took us out of the city, following the island's densely wooded spine. It reminded me of Ireland, with narrow roads under a canopy of trees. We visited a local *onsen* – it's obligatory for the tourist in Japan. The others couldn't wait to take their clothes off and dip into scented pools, full of loud Japanese families, all having noisy fun. Most male and female delegates veered off into the designated bathing sectors. They said they had to wash themselves before they bathed. Rows of naked men and women, busy with soap and shampoo and hairdriers. They slid their bodies into water that was warm and rich in healing minerals.

It didn't appeal to Tony or me. We sat together primly on a bench like fully-clothed survivors on an ice-floe after the Titanic disappeared beneath the waves. I was pleased he was there. I didn't feel as insular as usual.

We met in my room the night before the conference ended. Each country's delegates had to give a short exposition on the final day, to weave the threads of all we'd learned into a coherent fabric. We debated even the smallest detail. We reached a point when there was nothing we could add. Silence seeped like curdled milk into the space between us on the couch. Tony sipped his drink. I heard him swallow. The clink of ice sounded disproportionately loud and resonant against the crystal glass. I turned towards him and started to unbutton his shirt. Purely out of habit. My fingers did it of their own volition – it was their programmed response to silence. They were more conditioned than Pavlov's dogs.

It was a memorable evening.

I felt a wave of relief when he finally closed the door behind him. I always felt relieved when they left but this time there was an added dimension. Perhaps content would be a better choice of word. I felt the same sense of certainty as when I run a hot bath on a winter evening. Kate and I were reared on hot baths as a source of solace. My mother always said, 'I'll run you a nice hot bath', when we fought or failed or reached rock-bottom. It was like a mantra in our childhood.

Over the decades, I've developed a lot of faith in the efficacy of hot baths. I'm always freezing when I take my clothes off. I'm not comfortable with nudity, even on my own. I venture a foot and feel it start to warm. I slowly add myself, limb by limb, until the water overwhelms me, rippling and distorting the outline of my body. Warmth flows through me like a bloodstream. Things never seem so bad as I watch the steam rise off the water, misting the windows, softening the harshness of the current view.

I felt like that when Tony left my bedroom. The Oxford defines content as satisfaction. It's a term used in the House of Lords to indicate an affirmative vote. That's what Tony earned that night – a long term, affirmative vote. There was also an element of relief – that's defined as deliverance from anxiety. Redress of a grievance. I'd certainly been anxious. Without doubt, I felt aggrieved. I was the older sister, after all.

Everyone knew Kate would marry Michael. There was zero risk attached to that prediction. I was jealous. Not because I dreamed of clouds of tulle and satin flower-girls. Marriage as a concept wasn't the drawcard – it's defined as an intimate union for the procreation of lawful offspring. Neither intimacy nor offspring holds any appeal for me.

But people would feel sorry for me if my little sister married first. 'Poor Claire,' they'd say. Again. 'She's such a strange girl. So different from Kate. She'll probably be on her own forever.'

I was tired of being the lesser sister.

Tony and I had visited a holy shrine that afternoon. We walked through the structured garden, green with sculptured trees and beds of flowers. I knelt barefoot in the gold-encrusted temple. I remember the smell of burning incense, the hypnotic chanting of the brown-robed monk as he read the prayers of passing travellers. I heard a mellow gong. I wrote my prayer on a piece of paper and dropped it into the holy water at the entrance to the shrine. I watched it dissolve before my eyes.

The Japanese delivery ethic is remarkable. That very night the gods presented a solution. Tony would do, I thought.

Kate wouldn't beat me to the altar, after all.

Tony : Sepia. Background blended.

I've never been in love with Claire. Or anyone else. I couldn't even say I love my mother, despite the central role she's played. Love's not an active word in my vocabulary. I don't think I could define it if they asked me in a quiz. Perhaps it's what I feel for Amy. Value is a more familiar concept. I value Claire. I'm used to putting a price tag on assets — it's how I make my living.

I'd been with Irving Life for fifteen years when she joined the staff. I was on the panel when she came for the interview. As a formality. In deference to my position.

I make a measurable contribution to the balance sheet at Irving but I doubt whether they value my judgement on appointments. Human resources isn't my forte. I was a senior partner by then. This position was an integral part of my persona in my mother's eyes. She no longer introduced me merely as her son – she always said my son, senior partner at Irving Life. My job validated me in her eyes – and everybody else's, I suppose. The title made me harder to overlook. People had to take me seriously.

My subconscious recognised Claire's interview as a significant event. It's filed forever in my mind, in subtle shades of black and grey – it has the detailed clarity of a photograph in a catalogue. The long table – varnished wood, smooth and glossy to the touch. Smoke rising from Bernie's cigarette – a solitary rebellion against the regulations. My glasses lay on a sheaf of papers and caught the light that filtered through the blinds. A tall jug of icy water. A painting with glazed and clotted colours on the wall behind Claire's head. It's by George Boys – I've never related to it, despite its value. I've heard people say it's a technical triumph but I find it difficult to read. I prefer realistic landscapes of places I remember. That George Boys' painting is as ambiguous as Claire.

She made a good impression. We'd already seen the others on the shortlist – intelligent young men with old faces, conservative in pinstriped suits. Actuarial science doesn't appeal to incendiaries like Kate. Claire was a female clone of her predecessors. She was also in a pinstriped suit. Tailored trousers. A soft white shirt in Indian cotton. Cool and clinical. She could have been a surgeon. Her assured answers cut through the inquisition like a scalpel. Claire's intimidating.

But she's also stunning.

She takes your breath away. I noticed the gloss of her dark hair, caught in a shaft of sunlight. She looks more like a photographic model than an actuary, with her patrician profile and flawless skin. Her focused eyes seem out of place. They make you keep your distance. I couldn't look at her directly. My gaze shifted down. To her body. By mistake – I'm not an ogler. I felt even more uncomfortable than usual when I registered an impression. Long thighs. Breasts that make a statement, even under a pinstriped suit.

The competition didn't stand a chance.

Even my mother was impressed. She considered Claire good enough for me. Claire's never realised what an accolade that is. My mother is terminally myopic about her only son. Her version of me is diametrically opposed to common opinion. I've never had to validate her fantasy. She believed in me implicitly, in spite of all I failed to do. It's like Father Christmas – children believe in him because it's to their advantage. My mother's a clerk in the municipality. I am her only interest. My first class degree is her highest achievement. My job is her ultimate success. She thinks other people will be as dazzled as she is.

Claire's baffled by my relationship with my mother but she underestimates the effect of forty years. I'd hardly spent a night away from home before I married Claire – that's what made Tokyo such a landmark. Everyone at Irving was comatose with shock as they watched what happened when we got back.

Only my mother was not amazed by Claire's choice.

They all thought it was the money. I earn a lot of money. My income as a director is public knowledge – I make millions every year. But my mother didn't see it that way.

She thought the absence of women in my life was entirely due to my immersion in work. And to my exalted position in the company – no one dared aspire that high, in her opinion. Claire's beauty and intelligence gave her the necessary credentials. My mother thought Claire had recognised a kindred spirit.

I still don't understand why Claire's plans included me, why I became the focus of her attention. It's one of many things we don't discuss. Maybe Claire's never verbalised why she married me, even to herself. The marriage works and that's the important point. We're both more at home with results than reasons. That's where our approach to Amy is different from Kate's. She still agonises about why it happened.

Everything always comes back to Kate. She influences all Claire's decisions. She must have been a motivating factor in Claire's choice of marriage partner but I can't imagine why. Kate wouldn't have promoted me as a suitor. I made no impression on her at all. She struggled to remember my name at the outset.

Perhaps Claire only married me because her options were limited, in spite of all her assets. You have to be lacking a dimension to survive with Claire.

I fit all the specifications.

*

I was standing at the urinal when I first heard them talking about Claire.

'You'll never guess where I got lucky last night,' said Anderton, undoing his zip.

'Considering your current success rate, you probably had to resort to a hooker in Yeoville,' said Conroy. They were both young recruits on our accelerated executive advance programme.

'You couldn't be further from the truth,' he replied. 'It was none other than our very own ice maiden.'

'You mean Claire?' Conroy sounded incredulous. 'In your dreams perhaps,' he continued sceptically as he zipped up and turned to go.

'I'm telling you, it's true!' persisted Anderton. 'I wouldn't believe you either, if our roles were reversed. But she could hardly wait. Bloody strange girl, I must say. I was amazed that she agreed to come in the first place. And she didn't come on to me at all during dinner. It was heavy going – but when we got to her place . . .'

Their voices faded as they walked out. Conroy laughed as they turned the corner. He still sounded sceptical.

I didn't believe Anderton either. Exaggeration was a way of life for him. He already saw himself as an executive. I heard he didn't play to his handicap – no one wanted him in their team on a golf day. I'm surprised he wasn't sued for sexual harassment. He always stood close to the women when something came up for discussion. Right behind them, leaning forward on the desk. Arms touching. Double meanings and sexual innuendo were the trademarks of his conversation. Claire would never look at him. It was too incongruous. I was certain it was barroom fabrication – another Anderton ego trip.

I knew it was fantasy.

He said it again at the function before we left for Japan. He nudged me in the bar where I was standing, pretending to be part of the group.

'You could be onto a good thing here Tony! Don't underestimate your fellow traveller. You should aim for more than balance sheets next week . . .' He sniggered suggestively into his glass. Another nudge. I ignored him but it made me nervous. More nervous. I was already terrified at the prospect of a trip to such a foreign destination. The thought of small talk to Claire for the duration of the flight was daunting. What would I say? For all those hours . . .

I hate flying. Air travel has always made me sick. Physically sick. I've never seen anyone else use the bags they give you. Maybe it's the meals – they're disgusting. I hated the thought of an airport with as foreign a name as Tokyo. I was sick with anxiety that I'd get in the wrong queue. How would I find the hotel? I wouldn't be able to read the road signs. I wanted the trip to pass as quickly as possible. I wanted to get home. I'd never been on an international flight without my mother. She always organised everything. She had contingency plans for every possible scenario.

My earliest childhood memory is the day she left me at school for the first time. She'd never left me before. I felt as if I was drowning when I saw her walk away. I didn't cry because I thought it might make the others look at me – being the centre of attention is still my concept of hell's inferno. But my legs were shaking. I couldn't string words into a sentence to answer a question. Time stopped for me that day – that endless day. Break was the worst. I didn't know where to go. My mother had always been there to tell me where to go. We went everywhere together. And now she'd left me. I remember the welcome darkness of the shadow that hid me from invading eyes. I sat behind my tree, praying for a bell to ring, praying for the bell that would bring her back to fetch me.

She was the first mother there. Naturally. Her morning had been as fraught as mine. We were codependents. I should have been the child of an early pioneer where home schooling was the only option. But my mother wasn't pioneer material. There are risks involved in pioneering. You don't know what the future holds. My mother always knew exactly where she was going. She knew about the toilet facilities and the menu. Choice and chance are words she's eliminated from her vocabulary. After my father died, she couldn't contemplate the possibility of making another mistake.

But she made some sort of mistake with me. Despite her avalanche of good intentions, I never really moved forward from that first day at school. I've acquired impressive qualifications and a healthy bank account – but I don't function independently outside the office.

I've merely shifted my focus. Claire's my mentor now. I rely on her to make all our decisions.

*

I read *Sons and Lovers* as a set-book at university.

It struck a chord with me. I'm the archetypal mother's boy. I earned the label on that first abysmal day at school and I've never done anything to justify a different appellation. I'm not ignorant. I know all about Oedipus and his slaughtered father. I've studied Freud and his psychoanalytic theories but I don't agree with him. I've never seen myself as a clone of DH Lawrence. I remember a

31

letter Lawrence wrote, just prior to his mother's death. He said that he hated his father. He describes his parents' marriage as a carnal bloody fight. He'd been like one with his mother – but their relationship was more than filial and maternal. It had a husband and wife dimension. He spoke of a fusion of souls.

It wasn't as complicated as that for me. I didn't hate my father. The only way I knew him was through the tales my mother told me. I'd heard all about their courtship. Many times. It was one of my regular bedtime stories. Courtship is an old-fashioned word but it describes the relationship I picture between them. They both worked in the munici-pality. He was in the Accounts Department. She always pronounced it in capital letters. My mother was in awe of anyone who could add. I was just like my father, she told me with satisfaction.

When he died, I fitted perfectly onto the pedestal she'd built for him.

I was only a toddler at the time. He was a chronic diabetic – another thing we have in common. He went into a coma while she was away visiting her mother. The wrong dosage of insulin apparently – surprising for a man so skilled with figures. Hypoglycaemia. The level of his blood sugar plum-meted. The doctor told her he would have lost conscious-ness within a matter of minutes. And his heart was already weakened by the disease. She knew that.

But my mother shouldered responsibility for his death for the rest of her life. She was convinced it would never have happened if she hadn't gone away. She'd monitored his intake and his diet. She guessed he'd skipped some meals. Perhaps he'd taken a longer walk than usual – to pass the time without her. She poured through the medical textbooks in search of ways in which she could have failed him. Guilt was her paramount emotion. She never forgave herself. She tried to appease the gods through me. She wanted to assure them she'd learned her lesson.

She never let me out of her sight.

I didn't rebel against my overprotected situation. I liked it. I was never confronted with a decision. I valued the structure and security she gave me. Maslow's two primary needs are for sustenance and security. My mother provided a base as solid as the pyramids in this regard. I knew what time breakfast would be served. I knew exactly what would feature on the menu. I was absolutely certain that danger wouldn't penetrate the walls of our suburban home. My mother kept the windows shut. Net curtains held the world at bay. I felt totally secure at night as I lay beside her on my father's pillow and she pulled the blankets over us.

This is where I disagree with Freud. He interprets all memories as fantasies based on a child's sexual contact with his mother. He would have related all my inadequacies to my extended stay in my mother's bedroom. But there was no sexual agenda in my sleeping arrangements with my mother. It was purely a practicality. I never sleep through the night – a key symptom of diabetes is frequent urination. I have to get up several times a night. The toilet in my mother's house is adjacent to her bedroom. There's only one toilet. The other bedroom is at the end of a long corridor – it seemed a long, dark corridor when I was a little boy. I didn't like the dark. I felt safer with my mother.

And she slept better if I was close beside her. My father's death made her determined to be on call for me, twenty-four hours a day.

I was only seven years old when my diabetes manifested itself – juvenile diabetes is characterised by sudden onset. I still have a blurred recollection of the day it happened. My mother's reaction probably gave it stature in my memory bank. The premonitory symptoms are so familiar to me now. I know exactly what to do and so does Claire.

But that day, it was unexpected.

We were in a supermarket. Standing next to the breakfast cereals. I remember the boxes. Corn Flakes. Strawberry Pops. It's filed in the photographic recesses of my brain, alongside the one of Claire at her interview. I remember my sweaty palms. Feeling tired, although it was early in the day. I'd been in bed with flu – a viral infection can trigger the onset of a defect lurking in your DNA. Perhaps that's what happened to Amy. I remember the urgency of my mother's questions. Like bullets from a firing squad.

'What's the matter Tony? What's wrong?'

I don't remember what happened then. She said she picked me up. Rushed me to her doctor. Demanded immediate attention. I can imagine what a fuss she made. She's a low profile, long-suffering type of person – unless I'm the catalyst. She was gripped by an icy fear that it was going to happen again, that I'd slip away just like my father.

But diabetes is easily controlled with immediate attention. My recovery was almost instantaneous once the sugar solution slid into my veins. It didn't reassure my mother. There's no diabetic on the planet more strictly monitored than me.

My mother gave me my injection at precisely the same time every morning, before she poured our bedroom tea.

34

My diet was rigorously maintained. A careful calorie count to ensure optimum weight. My protein intake never fell below the requirement. No one in the accounts department at the municipality kept a more meticulous balance sheet than she did. Every result was stored in a logbook, filed in a cabinet in our hall. I'm sure my father would have been impressed. She had an armoury of diabetic tools. A blood glucose meter with a set of plastic strips. A set of visually read strips for urine ketones. Lancets, coated with sugar-sensitive chemicals – she'd whip one out and prick my finger. Glucose tablets. Her special carrying bag was geared for every emergency.

My health became my mother's life mission.

✳

My mother's obsessed with me. It obviously had an impact on my life but I wasn't unhappy with my lot. I felt secure and nurtured. I did well at school and university, in my solitary way. I don't resent her, despite the judgements Freud might pass on her approach to parenting. Freud's so negative. He believes human nature develops out of conflict and trauma and repressed anxiety. I don't regard his approach as scientific because he always works retrospectively. His conclusions on personality are based on a historical construction of what happened in the past. It's contrary to actuarial principles. I work out scientific formulae that deal with probable actions and predictable outcomes.

I focus on what's going to happen in the future.

I don't regard Freud's conclusions as valid. One of his disciples claimed that women hoard more pencils than men.

He linked it to penis envy. He saw pencils as phallic symbols. It's absurd. I admit that Claire hoards pencils. She has half a dozen in her handbag all the time – but she needs them to make her interminable lists. Statistically, women hoard more of every commodity than men. They don't specialise in phallic pencils.

I'm more an advocate of Alfred Adler. He also has a low regard for Eros and the pleasure principle. His theory starts with a helpless, dependent child – that's certainly part of my psyche. And Amy's. He claims everyone experiences feelings of inadequacy – develops specific lifeskills to help overcome them. His theory won't help Amy but perhaps it explains why I became an actuary. That specific lifeskill gives me credibility in the eyes of other people. In my professional role, I command respect. People ask my opinion. They value my judgement.

I get a completely different response if I meet someone at a cocktail party. Social events are not my forte. The outside world is not my forte. My house and my office are the only functional areas for me. I try to keep the time I spend in other venues to a minimum but some events are unavoidable. I have to see Claire's family sometimes. I dread it. An evening with Kate and Michael makes me revert to playground status. It's hard to believe that Claire and Kate are from the same genetic lineage.

Until you see Amy.

There's a large black and white photograph of the sisters in the entrance hall at their parents' house. They are totally unalike – and the photograph only gives a record of their physical appearance. Claire dominates that photograph. She overshadows Kate completely, with her cool patrician features, her elegance, her class. Kate's ugly. She looks as if she's from a different social stratum – a peasant girl beside the lady of the manor. Black and white photos throw everything into sharp relief. You can see the smudge of freckles on her cheeks. Her mouth's a careless slash. Disproportionately large. Almost garish. Her hair's unruly, tumbling on her shoulders. Claire's is smooth and dark, pulled back in a knot at the base of her neck.

The contrast between them couldn't be more extreme.

It's even more marked when you meet them outside that frozen moment. Claire doesn't change. She always looks like that, whatever the occasion, whatever she's wearing. She's remote. Unapproachable. The wounded would never turn to Claire for comfort.

She fades into the background when Kate walks into the room. Kate has an aura of energy around her. As if you've flicked the light switch and turned on a current. Kate's never neutral about anything. She agrees or disagrees. Emphatically. She laughs and cries with equal ease. Uses her hands to emphasise her point. She's always the focus of attention. I've seen her plait her arms round Michael's neck and kiss him. Anywhere. Whispering private secrets. I've also heard her shout and swear and lose her cool completely.

Claire and I never do that. Even if we're alone.

I'm sure I shrink in stature when I'm with Kate. I feel measurably smaller when she's in the room. Like someone turned to stone in Greek mythology. If I have to speak to Kate, I phone her. I'm more coherent with a cable length between us. I don't dislike her – no one could dislike her. But she's too warm for me. Too alive. She's vulnerable because she cares so much.

I find it easier to breathe when I'm with Claire.

Fortunately Claire seems almost as ill at ease with Kate and Michael as I am. Not that we've ever discussed it – but we're even quieter than usual on the way home after an evening when they're in the party. There's a sense of failure in the car. We can't raise enthusiasm for anything, whatever the proportions of the current crisis at work. We feel inadequate.

I noticed Kate and Michael exchanging glances at our wedding.

Neither Claire nor I wanted a church wedding. Our relationship progressed quietly on our return from Japan. We decided to get married, to tie up the ends. Neither of us likes an open-ended equation. A registry office during a lunch break would have suited us both. My mother was the problem. She was no more like Lawrence's mother than I was like him. She didn't resent Claire. She didn't feel her role usurped because I'd never been a surrogate husband for her. Claire's beautiful and successful so my mother saw her as another trophy for her display cabinet – someone to hang beside my certificates which lined the walls of the lounge.

Claire became another fixture in a house which served as a shrine to my achievements.

My mother insisted on a wedding exhibition for the other municipal clerks.

It was hardly an exhibition, although they were dazzled by the venue – the Westcliff is one of Johannesburg's top hotels. It wasn't a venue frequented by my mother's fellow workers. Or by her. Or by Claire's family. No one relaxed and let their hair down but it wasn't that sort of wedding.

We had a service at St Columba's because it's close to the Westcliff but it was far too big a church for our lean congregation. Claire didn't blunt her pencil preparing that particular list. We didn't know who to invite. Neither of us has throngs of friends. Neither of us has any friends.

We didn't want to ask people from work. No one at Irving Life could believe we were getting married. They wanted invitations merely because they were curious. We didn't want to give them any further cause for gossip so we didn't include them. We restricted the list to the municipal clerks and Claire's family. We filled barely three pews.

We had a luncheon on the balcony of the hotel. There was a string quartet and a view and that was virtually all the occasion had to offer. It was a quiet, low key event. No speeches – I had to draw the line somewhere. Some things are beyond me. Claire's mother tried hard – she circulated, talked to my mother and her friends. I've always liked Claire's mother because she makes an effort to include me. She invites my mother to tea and listens as she recites the catalogue of my achievements. She's more patient than Kate. Maybe it's because she loves Claire – she's delighted that it's worked for us.

Kate's wedding was completely different. As a social event, it would get a higher rating from every single person on the guest list – and it was a much bigger guest list. Everyone drove down to Cathedral Peak for the weekend. I must admit that the view from the tiny chapel window is superior to the Westcliff's. The basalt cliffs of the Drakensberg make more of a statement than suburban Johannesburg. Kate and Michael are addicted to the berg. They hike for days with rugged boots and heavy backpacks. I would never hike. I prefer an organised tour – you know what to expect. You can leave a detailed itinerary at work in case something comes up that needs your attention.

I wish something had come up the weekend of Kate's wedding. It was an ordeal for Claire and me.

Kate's friends are overwhelming. I don't think anyone's told them that the flower-children epoch ended in the sixties. They all wear funky clothes and smoke and drink and dance without any inhibitions. That's why Cathedral Peak is an ideal venue – everyone can get drunk or high without the threat of being arrested on the way home. They were all drunk that night. Even Claire's father was led off to bed. Claire and I were a tiny island of sobriety. It reminded me of our visit to the *onsen* in Japan. That was the first time I realised that Claire was a comfortable travelling companion.

I felt as if I was travelling with my mother.

My mother and I didn't travel much. She had no money while I was growing up. I wasn't allowed to go away on field trips at school. Thank goodness. Even a day trip in the school bus was an ordeal for me. I had no one to sit next to. I could hear them all laughing. I felt they were laughing at me. In retrospect, I realise that it wasn't like that. No one even noticed I was on the bus. If I hadn't been so punctual, they would have left without me – my absence wouldn't have been reported to the teacher.

I took my mother away on holiday when my salary began to reach astronomical proportions. She didn't like to be away for long because of the cat. We always went on a package tour – usually to the Oyster Box in Durban. It's an old fashioned hotel with courteous Indian waiters. She likes the menu. Soup and fish and a roast with three vegetables.

We were collected by a courier service and dropped at the airport. It's only a one-hour flight so I don't have to eat a meal. I don't have time to feel sick. We enjoyed our gentle excursions to Umhlanga.

Fortunately my job doesn't demand much travelling. I can deal with virtually everything on the Net. I had to go to London on occasion but I always took my mother with me. She monitored my insulin and we went on city tours to see the Tower of London and other attractions we'd heard of. We even saw some West End shows. She mounted all the photos in an album and took it to the office when we got home.

Japan was different. She was over sixty when the trip came up and the lengthy journey was too long for her to contemplate – her asthma had worsened by then. She was far too cautious to consider Japan a tourist venue – she would never leave her room in Tokyo. She and I were equally appalled at such a foreign prospect. She begged me not to go.

'What if you have a problem with your insulin?' she asked, anxiety in every syllable.

'They won't understand you. How will you explain to a doctor? Look what happened at Pearl Harbour,' she warned me.

Logic is not my mother's strongest suit.

I had to go. I was Claire's mentor. The AIDS model was critical, both to the company and on a national level. It incorporated all the most up to date information on the crisis. Claire and I had improved the fit to antenatal seroprevalence data and allowed for separate male and female assumptions. We covered trends in mortality, fertility and future migration. We allowed for bimodal paediatric HIV survival and various other technical innovations.

Claire was too junior to deliver the presentation without support although the major contribution to the project had been hers. She'd worked on it for her thesis. My role was to polish and improve, to anticipate possible queries from an international audience reticent about investment in Africa. It made no sense to send anyone but me. I was a senior partner with the relevant specialisation and skills.

I was forty-two years old. I couldn't admit that I was frightened.

I don't think I've ever been as frightened as that night when Claire started to unbutton my shirt. I felt the touch of her long, slight fingers. Like moths. They barely touched my skin. I'd had sexual fantasies, I suppose. Mild, unbidden fantasies with faceless, nameless women. I pushed them to the back of my subconscious. A woman's body existed only as a blurred outline in my mind. I shied away from specific detail. Nipples and pubic hair weren't in my vocabulary. Kate and Michael's standard sentence structure makes me wince – swearing's as intrinsic to them as punctuation. My nights in my mother's bed had been so chaste I'd never seen her out of her pyjamas.

I had no idea what Claire expected me to do.

Her fingers paused in surprise when they encountered the hard black plastic of the insulin pump I wore strapped around my waist. She looked in amazement at the slender syringe with its snake of fragile tubing, at the needle inserted underneath my skin. The insulin dripped slowly and continuously, keeping me stable.

I've never felt less stable than when she asked me softly

if she could take it off. I felt her fingers working on the buckle. It felt as if she was peeling away a layer of my skin. My body was in unprecedented turmoil.

I couldn't meet her eyes at breakfast next morning. I hadn't slept at all. I'd stared out of the window at the neon signs and small figures on the streets below my lofty view-point – I wasn't the only one awake in downtown Tokyo. I stood there all through the night.

I'm impotent.

I can imagine how Freud would rub his hands together and point fingers at my mother. He'd crow and say I told you so. He'd blame it all on my extended stay in my parents' marriage bed. But that's got nothing to do with my condition. Impotence is the only side effect of diabetes that my mother never discussed with me.

Claire and I have never discussed it either. I still have no idea why it doesn't seem to matter. And Amy's made it matter even less.

I'll always regard her as a rather complicated privilege.

*

A rather complicated privilege – perhaps Amy's not the only one who fits that description. I don't have a wide acquaintance but it seems true for all the sons and daughters who've featured in my life. Claire and Kate. Michael. Even for myself.

All our mothers might describe us in that way.

Diabetes is my particular complication from my mother's viewpoint. Because it killed my father, she regards the fact that I'm alive as a privilege. She's chronically anxious about my welfare but I've never seen her as flustered as the day I told her I'd invited someone from the office to have Sunday lunch with us at our house.

'Someone from the office?' she echoed. 'Sunday lunch?' She sounded a bit like Amy – except that her voice was loaded with emotion. I'm not surprised that she was disbelieving. It was the first time in over forty years that I'd invited someone to our home.

I was equally amazed by Claire's persistence. Our flight home had been an ordeal. With the AIDS model behind us, we'd run out of conversation. We no longer had a common interest. And my thoughts were swamped by recollections of the night before. Would she tell anyone? I flinched as I imagined how Anderton would snigger. Eyes following me as I walked down a corridor. Smirking. Ridicule.

It was a long, silent flight.

And now I'd invited her to lunch. Someone from the office. That's all she was at that stage. I was confused. What was she doing? What were her motives? First the seduction. Then the lack of gossip. An invitation to the theatre to watch her sister's play. Cappuccino after work in the coffee bar across the road. Although Claire didn't initiate it, office gossip started. A conversation stopped when I walked into the urinal – but it wasn't ridicule I sensed. It seemed almost akin to respect.

My relationship with Claire altered my standing at Irving Life.

My mother was thrown completely off balance by the lunch date suggestion. It wasn't only the prospect of a visitor. It was her gender. My mother had never considered the prospect of another woman in my life.

Claire altered her standing too.

I assured her that cold meat and a salad was all that was needed for the menu but she brushed me aside. I think the entire municipality was involved by the time the day arrived. For a week she sifted through the various recipes that had been suggested. She was up at dawn. Arranging flowers. Setting the table. Simmering the casserole. She dressed for the occasion — she looked as if she was setting out for church.

And church was the only place she wanted to go to after meeting Claire. To pray that she'd come again. To dream of wedding invitations for all the friends who'd come up with recipes. To imagine what they'd say when they saw the photos. I think she'd been expecting someone older. She'd probably thought along the lines of glasses and a bun. A younger version of herself . . .

She was bowled over by Claire's beauty.

She was worried about what she'd say to Claire — because she was an actuary. An exalted species in my mother's eyes. She was afraid she wouldn't understand the topics of conversation. But it didn't prove to be a problem — Claire hardly said a word all afternoon. She seemed content to listen to my mother. She sat through my life history. Juvenile diabetes. My student accolades. Step by step through my career . . .

My mother was in her element. The municipality had heard it all a million times. Claire was a brand new audience. She never anticipated that the afternoon would go so well. She didn't question why someone like Claire would opt for someone like me. All three mothers in my personal portfolio are myopic about their children. It's one of the few things they have in common.

Although they're both single mothers, addicted to an only son, Michael's mother and mine seem the most diametrically opposed. She looks like a reincarnation of Joan Baez. She wore jeans and a tie-dye T-shirt the afternoon Claire's mother invited us all to a family tea to celebrate our engagement. My mother wore her church outfit in honour of the occasion. She looked like a low-profile edition of the Queen Mother as they sat side by side on the sofa. She was outside her comfort zone. Overawed. Her life was circumspect. Home. Work. An outing to the shops. Umhlanga Rocks was the furthest she'd been. She was the only person in the room without a tertiary education. She was very nervous.

And so she talked incessantly. She launched her diabetes sermon. One paragraph flowed into the next. Juvenile diabetes. Sudden onset. Acidosis. Ketone bodies in the urine. Visual impairments. Hypoglycaemia. She was word-perfect with that particular script – but Michael's mother wasn't as tolerant an audience as Claire had been. She stepped into the breach as soon as my mother paused to take breath.

She wanted to deliver a speech of her own.

'My dear,' she began, leaning over to pat my mother's arm. It seemed an inoffensive opening but my ever-sensitive antennae went on red alert for nuance. Honed in on body language. I picked up a feeling of superiority. A patronising tone. I could feel my mother stiffen, even though we were divided by a coffee table and a stretch of carpet.

'What a coincidence!' she continued. 'This month's edition of *Astrology Today* arrived last week and there's a feature on medical astrology and diabetes. I think I've got it in my bag. I took it with me to the dentist because he always keeps me waiting.' She rummaged in the huge over-flowing basket that sat on the floor beside the small leather handbag I'd bought my mother on our last trip to London. 'Here it is!' she said triumphantly, pulling out a glossy magazine. 'Look at this!' she commanded as she spread the centrefold on my mother's lap.

It showed a complicated chart – it looked a bit like compass, with zodiac signs and a network of intervening lines. A miscellany of numbers. My mother might as well have been examining hieroglyphics on an Egyptian tomb-stone.

'This is the natal chart for a child with juvenile diabetes,' continued our astrological guru. She seemed determined to outshine my mother as an authority on diabetes – a sub-ject of no interest to anyone else. She pointed to a section of the chart. 'In diabetes, Venus rules the kidneys and a moon rules pancreatic action and blood flow. In this child's case, you can see a powerful post-natal solar eclipse – both natal and eclipse moon rule the stomach which explains why the child's diabetic. Did you have a natal chart drawn up for Tony?'

My mother looked blank. Defensive. 'I took him to the clinic. Every two weeks. He had all his injections . . .' she said, tentatively.

Michael came to her rescue. 'Oh shut up Ma,' he said lazily, lounging on the seat beside me. 'No one understands your bloody jargon! Can't you talk about the weather for a change?' My antennae picked up an air of sufferance. Kate had made him come against his will. Dragged him along to what promised to be a dreary afternoon. It seemed to go on forever.

His mother didn't shut up. She went on and on. My mother began to look anxious when she got on to chart indicators for the optimum approach to controlling diabetes. Something about mutability and worry overloading the digestive tract. I could almost hear my mother's thoughts tick over as she listened. She was starting to feel guilty. Maybe there was something she'd done wrong. She hardly said another word. She was out of her depth with Michael's mother. On another planet – that's probably a more apt analogy in the circumstances.

Claire's mother bustled between them, handing out tea and cake – eager for everyone to gel, to like each other, regardless of their differences. She had the same approach to Claire and Kate. Perhaps she was right – the gulfs between us don't seem insurmountable any more. Michael's mother had a lot of advice to offer about a theoretical child with diabetes but she hasn't come up with any answers in a real-life crisis. My mother's gained new stature with her contribution.

Amy levelled the playing fields.

Kate : Red. Multi-angled.

I grew up an only child.

I had a sister in the room next door but she might as well have lived in China. We spoke a different language. Claire was from Mars and I was from Venus – she left few footprints in my childhood memories. I can't say I actively disliked her – she was just there. She made no impact on my life at all. I had a closer relationship with the lounge furniture. There was a deep, soft, multi-cushioned couch next to the phone that was far more important to me than Claire. If the fireman offered me a choice between saving the couch or Claire, I'd have gone for the couch without a second thought. Even the phone would have taken preference. I relied a lot on the phone. I confided in it all the time so I had no need to talk to Claire. I've got friends who tell their sisters everything but it wasn't like that for us. We had no common ground. I was more in touch with my mother, despite the generation gap.

Things only changed because of Amy.

Claire's older than me. And significantly wiser. She doesn't share my propensity for rash decisions. That's why her decision about Amy shocked everyone who knew her. I didn't sacrifice anything for Amy. If anything, I've used her. Claire and I couldn't be more different despite everything we share today. Strangers are still surprised to hear we're sisters. Part of it's visual, of course. Claire's beautiful – dark and pale and sculpted. She reminds me of Vivien Leigh. She always looks cool, even in a heatwave.

There's only two years between us so we had concurrent school careers. The teachers always said, 'You're Claire's sister?', as if I was a major disappointment. Or perhaps a great relief. I can't imagine Claire making a contribution to classroom discussion. The maths teacher certainly preferred Claire. Mathematical concentration was a skill I never mastered. It seemed pointless to exert myself when my answers were inevitably wrong. I must have walked a million miles between the head's office and the maths classroom in my school career. Claire, on the other hand, was a mathematical genius. She could probably have given Einstein a few pointers. The maths department must have been terrified.

I used to read her school reports after everyone went to bed. I didn't look forward to the arrival of those long, white envelopes with their ominous crest. I was always grounded for life after they'd finished reading mine. Fortunately, my parents have short-term memories when it comes to school reports. A diplomatic kiss, a strategic cuddle, a fervent vow to turn over a new leaf in the future and they melted like a Christmas candle. Claire was never grounded after her report but she didn't sit on a pedestal and crow. She didn't seem to care. She was never elated, even if her maths mark was high enough to launch a choir of angels in a hallelujah chorus.

Claire's marks were oddly inconsistent – she was also good at grammar and music theory but her marks for literature and history were neutral. The only books I ever saw her read were set-books. And the fucking dictionary. What sort of maniac reads the dictionary? It's only one step up from the telephone directory. Claire was definitely from Mars. She would sit at the piano and play her scales for hours. Listening to her practise is my bleakest childhood memory. She played the same piece over and over again. Even the composer didn't play as accurately as Claire. I still flinch when I hear a piece from Claire's repertoire on the radio.

It's ironic that I'm involved with Michael, considering my deep-seated aversion to a keyboard. But Michael doesn't play like Claire. His music sucks you in, lifts you up. Claire's makes you keep your distance. She never played for anyone – not even for Granny and Gramps. They'd plead and beg. They were probably sick of sitting through my endless charades – I was addicted to charades. But Claire just shook her head. I don't think she played even for herself. She specialised in scales and disconnected bars. The piano teacher was the only one she aimed to please.

I'm completely different. I've never shunned the limelight. I love being centre stage. Recognition and acclaim are as necessary to me as breathing. Applause flows through my veins like a vital bloodstream. I'd die without it.

My stage career was launched with a nativity play in pre-school. It's probably my earliest coherent memory. I was cast as a cow in the stable. I had horns and a blanket. I was committed to my bovine role. I mooed around the house for days in preparation. I was as bad as Claire with her scales. My mooing on the night threatened to drown the Bible readings. There was a ripple of laughter from the audience. It was my first adrenaline rush. I wanted to break out of my background stall and climb in the crib with baby Jesus.

From that day onwards, I hankered after the leading role.

✳

I'm now a household name in the world of South African theatre – which means that the vast majority of the country's households have never heard of me. There aren't any theatres in Soweto and Khayelitsha – they aren't even on the drawing boards. Those are crammed with plans for schools and houses and hospitals. The budget in our fragile new democracy doesn't include luxuries like theatre.

It's not only in South Africa and the basket cases of the world – theatre's at risk everywhere in the new millennium with its webs and networks. The West End and Broadway are more a tourist attraction than the cornerstone of international theatre. It's the Changing of the Guards – Lloyd Webber and his rivals are the major drawcards now.

A large slice of the audience doesn't know that music isn't always part of a theatre excursion.

I've opted for a precarious profession.

But I had no choice. A theatre passion's like a runaway bush fire – once it's been ignited, it can't be deflected or extinguished. My fuse was lit in that lowly, pre-school stable and caused a fire that burned as strongly as Christianity for a crusader. Popcorn at the movies was never as exciting for me as the sawdust of a circus or the rollicking chorus at a pantomime.

Live performance! It's much more of an occasion than anything a screen can offer, regardless of size and special effects. I remember seeing *Equus* on stage – emotionally draining, despite the broomstick horses. An exposé of the violence of the human psyche. It's harrowing. And then I saw the movie. *Trouble in the stables* was the way one review described it. It's always so much less on screen. In my opinion anyway. And I'm always right about everything . . .

I spent my childhood dressing up. Pretending. My world was make-believe. Puppets and fairies far outranked adding up and spelling.

'It's such a lovely day darling – come outside and join us at the pool,' – my mother's weekend plea, as she peered into the darkened chaos of my bedroom, with its clutter of cardboard boxes. A makeshift stage, draped with sheets and towels. Painted cut-outs of trees and hillsides. An over-flowing costume cupboard – cast-offs to clothe anyone from a princess to an orphan. A miscellany of ancient make-up jars, piled at random by the mirror. The crown jewels, scattered on a messy table. A clutter of props – from a broomstick to a broken china tea set. Vital possessions. I was always at work on a new production.

It wasn't an ideal scenario. I didn't want to act out my fantasies in private. I craved an audience. I wanted to go public with my thoughts and feelings. I needed applause and recognition but it wasn't easy to come by. My parents were at work. My friends preferred the pool. And Claire was always practising her fucking scales. I usually had to settle for Agnes – our luckless maid, assigned to clean my bedroom. It was such a daunting task that she was easily persuaded to sit down and watch the show instead. She thought I was wonderful. She fed my ego and fuelled my ambitions.

I'll always be in debt to Agnes.

And to Prof Rankin. He was the head of the Drama School at Wits when I applied. Short, bright, sardonic. Iron grey hair, tied back in a tail on his neck. At our initial interview, I tried to steer the conversation away from the matric certificate lurking in my handbag. It wasn't the sort of thing you'd like to bring out into the open. The symbols looked better in total darkness. Daylight would destroy my chances.

But Prof Rankin listened as I described my ruling passion. He looked through my portfolio. School productions. Local drama school. Modern dancing. A reference from my drama teacher. Some good reviews. He agreed to overlook my sagging symbols. Conditional acceptance – dependent on mid-year results. I was hard put not to leap across the table to embrace him.

I was desperate for my application to be accepted.

The staff at the Drama School was composed of a variety of high-ranking professionals – actors, designers, scriptwriters and directors. I loved everything about my course. Performance – voice, movement and acting. Improvisation technique. Physical theatre. TV and film studies. I even went to lectures and passed exams. I was involved in multiple productions – either on the set or in the cast. I remember the auditions, the long hours – even the boredom. The rehearsals went on forever – especially in a workshop. It's hard work unpacking a script. No one discouraged us from trying out a radical idea. Some were ghastly failures. I remember long, rueful post-mortems at the theatre coffee shop. I drank gallons of black coffee during my university career. The four years passed in a blur.

Claire was finishing actuarial science at the time, but the faculties are miles apart at Wits. And the ethos is totally different. Drama and Business Science are diametrically opposed. Claire and I had to share a car but it worked all right because our hours were so different. Claire didn't need the car at night. She had a steady stream of escorts who called to take her out. I never got to know any of them because I was always at the theatre. My parents were in a constant state of apprehension – Wits is an inner city university and the streets of Braamfontein aren't an ideal location for a girl on her own in the early hours of the morning. Michael was studying music at the Tech in Pretoria so he was seldom available as an escort.

But I survived. I was rapturously happy at university. I built long-term alliances with my fellow students. We wore funky clothes with wild hair and loud opinions. We thought we were infinitely superior to the Business Science squad with its brains and long-term focus. I cringe when I recall the arrogance of my student days. I was invincible at seventeen.

My big break came in my final year. Prof Rankin is a leading director in Gauteng. He came in for a lot of criticism when he cast me in the leading role for a mainstream production at the Grahamstown Festival that year. He decided to do *Master Class* – Terence McNally's tribute to Maria Callas. I became obsessed with Callas. Consummate artist. Legendary diva. I immersed myself in her passions and insights. I lived with her through her heady days at La Scala. I even fell in love with Onassis. It's an inspiring play to be a part of – I learned about love and joy and sorrow. What it takes to produce glorious art. What it means to be alive.

The opening night is engraved in stone in my memory. As permanent as the pyramids.

I was terribly nervous as I paced my dressing room. It was filled with flowers. From my parents. From Michael. Even from Claire. I knew they were all out there, dressed up for the occasion – part of the glamour of a first night audience. I'd stuck all the cards around my mirror. And there was a copy of the poster on the wall. *Master Class* in bold capitals – and underneath, my name and photo! I could scarcely believe it was true.

I forced myself to stick to my routine. Green tea. A protein dinner. A vocal warm up. Stretching. Music and a candle – one of those aromatherapy candles. They're supposed to have a calming influence but it didn't work. My stomach churned when the cue light came on and I moved towards the wings.

I've still got the review from that first evening.

New Talent at the Festival.

Rankin's gamble with an unknown student paid off when Master Class opened at the festival last night. Kate Templeton IS Callas.

She's sublime and devastating as La Diva. She carries her audience to the brink of ecstasy and despair, with an emotional repertoire unexpected in so young a performer. This is theatre. This is opera. If you see nothing else at the festival this year, don't miss Kate Templeton in Master Class.

My career took off after *Master Class* – as much as a career in South African theatre can be considered to have taken off. It's not a major galaxy in the theatrical world – not many night skies where a new star can find a place to shine and light the heavens. It's like a fucking black hole most of the time.

When I shook his hand at graduation, Prof Rankin gave me a valid warning. 'I know you want to be a commercial actress Kate,' he told me, in his wise and patient way. 'And you will be. You've got the talent and the motivation and that's a winning combination. But it's not enough. It's a tough, competitive profession. Even in London, they struggle to put on Shakespeare – the cast's too big. No one's got money any more. You have to have more than one string to your bow. You can't focus only on the stage. Try corporate theatre. Education. Don't knock the soaps – they'll make your name familiar to a wider audience than the theatre. Maximum flexibility – that's what's necessary if you're planning to stay solvent.'

He was right. It's been a roller-coaster ride for me and Michael. We're either rich or poor. Relatively rich. Comprehensively poor. My luckless parents still dig into their pockets and bail us out from time to time. Thank God Claire's around to lift their spirits.

But I wouldn't exchange my skills for hers. She and Tony seem to live a passionless existence, wired up to a world that's distant. They're closer to their email contacts in the States than to me and Michael – even though we have faces and a physical address. Claire and Tony only have websites on their visiting list.

But Claire and I have always had a lot in common though I didn't recognise it at the time. Both our jobs demand communication that differs from a normal conversation. Claire's armed with a mouse that puts her in contact with a host of strangers she'll never meet in person. It's an exchange of information. Solitary. It seemed so different to a stage performance – that's a shared experience, an outpouring of emotion.

But I never meet my audience. They're all strangers. Maybe we're not so different after all.

✳

We invited Claire and her new acquisition to dinner once they'd officially declared themselves an item. Mom asked us to and I'd do anything for her. She was delighted that Claire appeared to be involved in a relationship. At last. Claire wasn't short of dates but she'd never had a steady boyfriend. I think my mother would have welcomed Blackbeard the Pirate with a fanfare. Personally, I'd have been happier with Blackbeard but I didn't have the heart to tell her. At least Blackbeard might have had something interesting to say.

My mother could have invented the card game *Happy Families*. She'd never completely shelved her hopes that Claire and I would bond. She nourished visions of hordes of grandchildren clambering on her knees while her two daughters whipped up a salad in the kitchen, gossiping and sharing secrets.

Poor Mom. Dreams are dangerous commodities. They seldom deliver.

To get back to the dinner – it was a fucking disaster. Culinary skills are another of the issues that divide Claire and me. She's a gourmet cook. The meals I've had at her place are always daunting, both in quality and presentation. She favours nouvelle cuisine. We were always starving when we left.

Fortunately, they were rare occasions.

Anyway, I promised my mother I'd have them round. I made Michael comb his hair and change out of his tracksuit. I laboured for hours preparing a meal. It was up to my usual squalid standards. Lukewarm soup and a pasta dish – it looked like someone had thrown up in the serving bowl. Even Michael approached it with caution. But it wasn't the food that made the evening so awful – it was the conversation. They should put paratroopers through an evening like that. It'd show up those with the capacity for endurance.

'What does an actuary do, for Christ's sake?' Michael grumbled when I tried to give him guidelines for the night that lay ahead.

'It's sort of financial,' I said vaguely. 'Just talk about money. Or banking.'

That's risky for Michael. Anything to do with banks is a minefield. We're always overdrawn. Accounts go missing. Finances aren't his forte.

We limped laboriously through pre-dinner drinks. As another silence fell, I decided to get the meal on the table earlier than I planned. I left Michael to hold the fort as I went to the kitchen to apply the finishing touches. I could hear him searching for a topic as I eavesdropped from the kitchen.

'How are you financial gurus planning to stop the rand from falling any further?' he asked in a flood of inspiration. 'I'm beginning to feel I've seen my last West End show. It's getting harder than ever to justify a London jaunt.' It sounded a promising start from where I stood at the stove, feverishly stirring the pasta. I was praying it would miraculously transform itself into something edible. And Tony did brighten up, to some extent. He looked almost half-alive.

'Well, er . . .' he began. Most of his sentences started like that. Hesitant. Uncertain. As if he had no idea of the answer. In stark contrast to his fluency once he found himself on familiar ground – he then sounded as if he was reciting a textbook. 'We've just got the new review from the Free Market Foundation,' he continued. 'More and more countries are fixing the value of their currency to the dollar. Rather than depending on the continued favourable performance of any single benchmark currency, there could be significant benefit from diversifying to create a hybrid standard to which the local currency could be fixed.'

Michael looked bemused. Understandably. But Claire seemed to get whatever point he was making. The economy was more her scene than small talk. She and Tony probably chat about it over morning tea.

'But won't you end up with a basket of currencies or commodities – or both?' she asked him. 'I think it could just lead to over-diversification – surely it'd be less transparent and more difficult to monitor?'

'Maybe you're right,' mused Tony. 'I think they should rather choose two or three components – like the US dollar, the euro and a specified weight of gold. I think a ratio of 40: 40: 20 would be valid. The reserve bank could use a very simple formula to calculate the rand's value for monetary policy purposes – they could assess whether the rand was over or underinflated and buy and sell to control the quantity of rands in circulation.'

'Would anyone like some peanuts?' said Michael, glaring accusingly towards the kitchen. I felt the onset of mild hysteria as I sniggered over the pasta which wasn't responding to treatment. It was terminally ill.

Like the evening . . .

'Jesus, Kate,' hissed Michael as he snarled past me towards the dishwasher, laden with half-finished bowls of soup. 'This is fucking awful. Get rid of them. And what the hell happened to the soup? Why didn't you heat it up? What were those things floating in it?'

'Those were prawns,' I said coldly. I'd made a special effort with the soup.

'Prawns?' said Michael, disbelievingly. 'They didn't look like prawns. Mine looked more like a baby toad. I think some of them were still alive. I saw one poor bastard trying to make it to the edge . . .'

I ignored him. They were prawns – it said so on the packet. It would have been safer to buy a bloody tin of soup but I'd promised my mother a special event – to make dear Tony welcome. I had to admit I'd failed when she phoned at dawn for a report back.

'You've got to face it,' I told her. 'Claire and I are never going to gel. And Michael and Tony aren't even in the same galaxy. It was absolutely dreadful.'

Panic drifted down the phone line.

'No.' I reassured her. 'I'm not saying he's awful. It's just that he's so fucking boring. He's even worse than Claire. She's not the liveliest person on the planet but she's a laugh a minute compared to this guy. I don't think he can laugh. He might be able to measure the success of a joke on some statistical barometer but I can't imagine him ever laughing at one. But I think Claire likes him – as much as she likes anyone. They weren't exactly fawning all over each other but Claire's always like the bloody sphinx. I'm not having them again. It was worse than a fucking board meeting.'

Poor Mom. She was so disappointed that her bonding exercise had failed. It would take more than prawn chowder to bring Claire and I together. None of us could have predicted the formula we'd have to use.

It made the Reserve Bank's tactics with the currency look like child's play.

＊

I've always regarded myself as sensitive. Liberal. Open-minded. Democratic. I'd never vote Republican if I lived in America – I'm anti big business. I couldn't contemplate a corporate environment like Claire's, even if it earned me millions every year. Especially if it earned me millions every year. I glamorise our precarious budget – living on the edge, I call it. Our lounge is a hotchpotch of non-matching items but I tell myself it's warm and vibrant. I've given it a mental upgrade despite my secret knowledge that I'm merely too lazy to tidy up the mess. I hate Claire's antiseptic town house with its glass and chrome and leather.

When I look back on everything that's happened, I know my enlightened outlook has some very shady corners. I pass judgement on anyone who disagrees. My opinions are as cast in stone as those of a right-wing politician. That was one of my problems with Amy. Claire approached her, armed with reams of paper. Multiple suggestions. This is the information age and you can download an Amy-update on an almost daily basis. But I never research the conclusions I come to. I ignored everything Claire and Tony told me because I knew my own conclusions were the right ones. I favour emotion above fact when forming an opinion – and I've always had a glut of emotions at my disposal.

One of my many cast-iron opinions is that acting is superior to actuarial science as a career or lifestyle. This was a truth as fundamental as the sun rising daily in the east – despite the fact that I still have no idea what either Claire or Tony actually do. I know they disappear into an office skyscraper in the early hours of the morning and emerge in the early evening. I'm seldom coherent before mid-morning. Michael doesn't own a suit or tie.

I judged Claire and Tony according to these criteria and, of course, they failed my test. I wrote them off entirely – but I didn't want them to do the same to me. I wanted Claire to join the queue that lined up to watch me as I climbed the ladder into the national theatre spotlight.

'But Claire always supports you,' protested my mother. 'She never misses anything you're in. Even if it's in Cape Town. And Tony usually goes with her. If anything, you and Michael are more at fault than they are. Neither of you ever shows the faintest interest in actuarial models.'

'You can't compare actuarial models to the theatre!' I stormed. 'No one who's vaguely normal is interested in actuarial models. It's like curling up beside a fire in winter to read Stephen Hawking. Or James Joyce. Or the fucking dictionary, in Claire's case. The entertainment factor's zero. I've never seen her enjoy herself.'

When I was pissed off with Claire, I never got any support from my parents. I can't believe she didn't drive them mad but loyalty was a parental ethic in our family. They sat defiantly through all the parents' meetings when my sins were catalogued by assorted teachers. They never stopped applauding when I stepped forward to take a bow. They were terminally myopic when it came to family. Even Amy. Unconditional love is our family motto.

Not for me though. I have more stringent conditions. It wasn't enough for me that Claire pitched up to see my shows. It didn't feel like support. It felt more like criticism because she never passed a comment. She didn't say she'd enjoyed it, that I'd been convincing, that I'd made her laugh or made her cry – she never even said she'd been to see it. Maybe unconditional attendance is her version of the family motto. She never bunked school or piano lessons either but she didn't seem committed to them. She just went through the motions. School and piano lessons featured on her list of things to do each day.

Going to watch me in a show seemed to be like buying milk or eggs on her grocery list – a boring essential to be ticked off and packed into the trolley. But I wanted to be a carton of cream. A delicious luxury. Something to savour and remember.

I wanted Claire to praise me.

'But darling, you know what Claire's like,' continued her maternal support base. 'It's hard for her to show her feelings. She doesn't find compliments easy. Or criticism. But that doesn't mean she doesn't think you're good. That's why she goes to watch you.'

My mother was wasted as a housewife. If she'd been more ambitious, she could have carved out a major career as a diplomat in the United Nations. I'm sure she'd have got a nomination for the Peace Prize. Living with her daughters must have been more challenging than the Middle East or Ireland.

'God knows why she goes,' I snarled. 'She doesn't like theatre. She doesn't even like movies. She certainly doesn't like me. Why the hell does she bother to pitch at all?'

'You must stick to being an actress darling,' said my mother, as tartly as her unconditional credo would allow. 'You'd be the sort of psychiatrist I hate. You're always trying to find the answers and apportion blame for things that are different from the way you want them. Sometimes you just have to accept things as they are and move forward from there.'

She said that about Amy too but I still wasn't listening.

My mother and I were talking about *The Vagina Monologues* on that occasion. It's a demanding piece to do in South Africa. Vagina and cunt aren't words that come up often in our conversation. Especially one with Claire. I doubt if she has either. Bodily secretions aren't a concept I associate with her. Not even run-of-the-mill secretions like blood, sweat and tears. I've hardly ever seen Claire cry. It's imposs-ible to imagine her having sex. Particularly with Tony. Sex with Tony must be even more boring than a conversation with Tony – though it's hard to imagine anything more boring than that.

No critic ever says the *Monologues* is a boring play. It's not a cerebral piece where the audience sits in thoughtful silence. They're silent sometimes but it's always loaded with emotion. And they laugh. The success of the whole thing hangs on audience participation. That particular performance had gone particularly well. You can't guarantee the same rapport with every audience but it was good that night. I could feel they were all with me as they stood in noisy enthusiasm as I ended. I was flushed and drained as I stepped forward, warmth wrapping me like a blanket.

Then I noticed a woman on her own at the end of the row, right at the back. She was the only one still sitting. Not clapping. I saw her rise and fade into the exit.

It was Claire.

My warm blanket felt as if it had been wrenched aside, replaced by icy water and a freezing draught of air. I felt cold and naked and exposed. I told myself I didn't care as I sat backstage, scrubbing off my make-up. But I'm not as neutral about Claire as I claim to be. My mother has a large framed photo of us both in the entrance hall. Every single person who comes to the house stops and looks at it. And every single fucking person says how beautiful Claire is.

I wish there was something about me she envied.

Not even Michael knows that – and no one's closer to me than he is.

✳

Michael and I never had sex. Not before the eighteenth of November.

It seems ludicrous to make a claim like that about people as tactile as we are. Neither of us ever merely says hello. There's always a hug. Kisses. Our bodies contribute as much to a conversation as our words do. We use our hands for emphasis and punctuation – we're both very emphatic. We know everything. There are no neutral topics as far as we're concerned. It's almost as if we're bilingual. Multilingual. Body language is our second tongue. French. Italians. Spaniards – they can all understand our questions just by watching.

Our family genes are more evenly distributed with regard to bodies than they are to faces. My body is as good as Claire's. She doesn't deserve hers. Or her face, for that matter. She's made no use of either. She's always out of sight in a low-profile, tenth-floor office. She should have been slinking down a catwalk. Striking poses for the camera. I can't believe that someone with her potential has ended up with Tony. Lacklustre Tony. He could never have expected anyone to look in his direction. Especially someone who looks like Claire. It must have felt like divine intervention on the road to Damascus.

Michael's different. Everyone looks in his direction.

The first thing I noticed was his body. His face was obscured by the make-up. Red pouting lips. Garish cheek bones. Outlandish eyes and untamed hair. Arresting – but still overshadowed by his body. Hot-groin strutting. Pelvic thrusting. Leather coated like a second skin. His never-ending legs. High heels. Black stockings and suspenders . . .

My sweet transvestite. Transexual Transylvanian. Dr

Frank 'n Furter . . .

Michael became a legend overnight when the new drama teacher dared to stage *Rocky Horror* as the annual school production. I joined the queue of girls who thought he was the top prize that the school had on offer.

It was my first year at high school. As a well established legend, Michael wasn't available to someone in my junior league. He moved in celestial circles. He could have anyone he wanted. I had no qualifications for attracting his attention but I've always been ambitious. We sat in groups of girls, dreaming in circles – of boys and sex and possibilities . . .

We were transfixed when he and his friends gatecrashed the party – a squad of arch-angels down from heaven for the evening. Muffled shrieks. It's him. They dared me. Clustered whispers. Ask him. I downed my drink. Turned up the music. I walked over to his group and pulled him in among the other dancers.

Michael and I dance well together. Exhibitionist. Aware of people watching. We fitted like a jigsaw as our hands touched and our bodies grew familiar. We had more in common than I ever dared to hope.

I'm sure my hand tingled when I took his arm that evening. A current flowed between us. As if someone switched the lights on. I didn't place a high enough value on the experience at the time. I was only fifteen – I knew nothing about electricity. I thought it was the same for everyone. I was older when I learned that lights can go out. I'm sure that Claire and Tony live a life that's only lit by candles. Perhaps it's safer.

Michael's mother is Bohemian so we had early access to a bedroom. I love Michael's hands. His long fingers. His skin is smooth. Always tanned. I'm still crazy about him. He makes my heart turn over. He makes me laugh. He's an entertainer off the stage as well – more experienced than me in every type of entertainment at the outset. I had zero experience but learned quickly. The physical component was a major part of our new relationship but I never thought of it as having sex. We were always making love. We were intimate. *Intimacy* – I saw the film version of that novel. There it's only sex. No questions asked. No conversations. They're never intimate, despite the many ways their bodies merge.

Michael and I were different. For a while, anyway.

The way we were.

That's one of Michael's numbers. I can't listen to it now. It's the saddest song I've ever heard. Sex was all we had left after the eighteenth of November.

I sometimes wonder if I've an unrealistic recollection of those early years – all our starry nights. We seemed more in love than anybody else – as if we were the only ones alive in three dimensions. Some people do have more capacity for love. I've never believed all men are equal. It's obviously nonsense. Most people are average. They've got average jobs and average kids and average infidelities.

I thought Tony's mother epitomised the average concept – the municipal clerk with her glasses and her sensible shoes. Neat, carefully buttoned blouses. And my own parents seemed ordinary. My mother's a housewife who does temp work on occasion to swell the family budget. My father has an average job. In an office. Two weeks paid leave a year. They're vaguely religious. They love their parents and their friends. And their children.

69

But neither of their children is average.

Claire and Tony aren't like us but they're certainly not average. Both have skills beyond the norm. And they're strangely intimate, despite their distance. There are dimensions in that marriage I can't quite put my finger on. Maybe they lack a dimension. Or maybe they've got something extra. I know they aren't average.

And no one would ever say Michael was average. Or me. We both stand out. I'm not trying to rate us on a scale of superhumans. I'm not saying we're better than the rest. We've more faults than most. Many more. We don't merely make the odd mistake – we cock-up on a monumental basis.

But we're certainly not average.

Claire likes lists. I can imagine her drawing up a list, comparing sibling vice and virtue. Our vices would overshadow theirs completely. We're sloppy, sulky, angry. Loud. Drunk. Unreasonable. Michael's redeeming feature is his music – that's what makes him a cut above the rest. It flows through his arteries and his veins. It's more significant than blood. And not only his voice. Keyboard. Saxophone. Clarinet. Guitar. He's mastered them all. Magic fingers, like a wizard. No wonder they turn the heat up when I become their focus.

But it's more than musical ability. Claire's also musical. Exceptionally so. But their response to music is different. Michael wants to share it. He's a performer, playing to the crowd, milking every nuance. He has an eclectic repertoire. It goes beyond Lloyd Webber and Broadway blockbusters.

Because of his mother.

She's a flowerchild. A qualified astrologist. She lives by omens. She was a star-crossed lover – his father rode off into the sunset, leaving them to struggle in Bohemian disorder. They were vegetarian – naturally. Candles and incense. She was weird. I loved her when I was a schoolgirl, chafing against the deadlines of my respectable, suburban family unit.

Her doctorate focused on the creation myths of the bushmen – primitive astrological data, passed down orally through generations to explain their past and predict the future. Michael grew up with a backpack, hiking in the mountains and the arid wastelands, following the clues encoded in their paintings. Ancient bushmen lullabies threaded through his compositions. Haunting. Mystical. He dreamed of Johnny Clegg and the international spotlight. And so did I.

Until Amy. She narrowed everyone's choices.

She's not average either.

That's the equation – four non-average adults and their mutual child. No one knows how to work out the answer.

*

I think each of us made a conscious decision not to have children. It's not the sort of topic we'd discuss with Claire and Tony but I don't think they like children. Children are naturally intimate, with their clinging arms and sticky kisses. They attach themselves to your life like barnacles. They demand that you tailor it to them – it would be anathema to isolationists like my sister and the man she selected as her soulmate.

Children are also anathema to us. Michael and I are focused on ourselves. Our lives may be linked by the spotlight but it never shines on the same stage. I never audition for a musical. Michael's only a spectator at a play. We have separate lives, despite our passion for each other. Our individual space is valuable. We didn't want it invaded by a child.

Children stuff up your mobility completely. They like routine. Regular meals. Nutritious meals – not bread and yoghurt and pizza from the deli on the corner. Children mean you have to be frugal with your money. Make provision for their education. Saving wasn't a lifeskill Michael and I aspired to. The only goal we ever saved for was a plane ticket – then we'd blow the lot in London. Or in leafy Paris. We loved New York. Fifth Avenue and Broadway, alive with neon signs and yellow taxis. We also liked the fringe. Faded theatres that spoke of the past – and the future. We'd track down an offbeat performance – something innovative and daring that wouldn't make it in a mainstream location. The cutting edge of theatre.

Michael and I are extremists. Although the crowds are thrilling, we also like silence. The Drakensberg's the most silent place on earth – despite the birds and the wind and the sound of water. If we couldn't save the airfare – and we often couldn't – we opted for the berg. We were stalwarts of the mountain club at school. A weekend break away from home – away from supervision. A chance for sex at leisure. I always associate the berg with sex.

I think Amy was conceived there. I choose to believe it although I can't be certain it's true. I'm far too slapdash to back my theory with medical evidence. I've never tracked ovulation with a thermometer and stopwatch. I hoped I'd never ovulate at all. The last thing that I wanted was a baby.

We'd chosen Lesotho for the weekend when I think it happened. It's an ideal venue, if solitude is what you're after. Access is difficult. The skyline features three stark peaks. Inversed reflections as we strode out along the banks of the Tsoelike, with its minnows flashing just below the surface of the water. Overhead, a lammergeyer soared against the blue sky where the clouds were building.

It's totally isolated. There's no mountain rescue team so no one knew we were stranded. We'd followed a pebbled footpath, winding upwards. The park is rich in rock art – Michael's mother's speciality. Before we left, she'd reminded him of an earlier hike they'd done. He was determined to track the paintings down. He tackled the task with the same enthusiasm he showed when hunting down a backstreet theatre in a Broadway alley. I pointed out that the clouds were mounting but Michael's difficult to deflect in tracker mode.

'We're nearly there,' he told me.

We reached the overhang moments before the sky was split by lightning.

'We're going to die of exposure,' I snarled as we huddled together bleakly, damp and insecure against the onslaught of the rain. 'It's your bloody mother's fault. Why she had to mention the fucking paintings . . .'

'Kate. Katie,' said Michael, smiling at me through the rain. Kissing my wet cheeks, my rat-tail strands. 'It won't last. You're always so Learish. Taking on the elements. Ranting and raving. You look bloody sexy in a wet T-shirt . . .'

He pulled me towards him. 'Relax. It'll be over soon . . .'

And it was. The weak sun crept back onto our mountain

canvas – but limp and ineffectual. Not enough to daunt the water, flowing strongly downhill. Loaded with mud. Treacherous, even in thick-soled shoes . . .

'We'll have to spend the night here,' said Michael, searching in the distant angles of the cave. Miraculously, he found a cache of wood – a pile of sticks and branches, untouched by the storm. We coaxed a fire to life and warmed our hands as it flickered. We could see the enigmatic figures, painted on the walls before the start of history.

'Look at the colours,' said Michael, quoting the maternal oracle responsible for our damp and isolated predicament. 'Ochreous earth. Ground up mineral oxides and coloured stones. They mixed it with animal fat. Milk and honey. Ox-blood. Urine. Bird shit. I'm always amazed by the varied palette they came up with.'

The pictures looked eerie, their colours haunting in the firelight. A vermilion smudge, merging into orange. White and charcoal. Mythical creatures – half mantis, half man. Fish figures, human to the waist. Elongated hunters. Eland in polychrome. They faded into darkness as the wood ran out and we fell asleep, zipped up tight against the mountain chill.

It was still cold when the sun surprised us with an early wake-up call. We folded defensively together. Warming quickly. Temperatures rising faster than the frosted air around us. I remember the birds and the sound of breathing – but it still seemed profoundly silent.

I like to think that Amy started then.

Amy. Our sea-change child. Elusive. Alien. Our girl from the Far Away Tree.

We made love that morning. In a cave. Cut off from

other people by strands of curling mist. Strange figures on the background walls. Filtered light and shadows . . .

A dreamscape – the perfect background set for Amy.

Amy : Circular. Colour-coded.

Microscopic, barely visible, heavy with potential, the ripened ovum starts its journey. As it travels, a swarm of cells clusters round it, programmed to feed and nurture. A tadpole tide strikes upstream to meet it on a route mapped out at the start of human history.

Convergence.

A mosaic of interlocking molecules blocks the way. Tentative survivors of the journey probe into a reef of coral membrane, guardian of the core. A solitary sperm persists, burrowing through the barrier, sucked into the softness.

Fusion. A new beginning.

Amy . . .

My cell shimmers, translucent, out of sight — a strange sea creature from the ocean's deepest reaches. Packaged at my core are chromosomes — twenty-three that link me to my father — and another twenty-three, my mother's contribution. Strands of DNA. The double helix. Genetic instructions that dictate my future.

My cell splits into two. And into four. And eight. Division and replication. Multiplication. I'm a blackberry of clustered cells — a silver shimmer, rolling inexorably towards my target. The lining thickens, aware of the imminence of my arrival. I anchor myself, extending tendrils. I'm rooted and I start to grow. I'm one month old . . . a sprouting bean. Tissue-paper skin, a pulsing heart-beat, sea-horse ridges down my spine. Budding arms and legs, fringed with toes and reaching fingers. My brain — a tangle of neurons and electrical impulses, building — outward, upward and inward — assigning duties, making order out of chaos.

At five weeks, my brain's unstructured — then fully wired in less than forty days. I'm vulnerable then. The enemy's an alien. A virus, targeting a group of genes mutated from my mother — no more than ten. It's a tiny number compared to the billions more I have at my disposal. They're unstable genes and prone to rearrangement. They've got power over other genes. They turn them off. Or on. No one sees them. No one can stop them.

They undermine my future.

I'm six months old. I stretch my arms. I kick my feet. I'm a fish in a warm balloon of water. I drink and suck, my fingers curled like fronds in a seaside rock pool. I feel the wetness of the water, my white creamy skin. I'm growing —

curled in a tight ball, knees under my chin, my head pushed forward on my chest, arms crossed in front. I hear my mother's voice. My eyes are open. I'm aware of dark and light. I take a step. I'm ready . . .

They think I'm perfect when they see me. I cry on cue. I move my arms and legs. My fingers and my toes both add up to ten. Their specialists tick all the columns on their rating scale. They won't find out. None of the tests they run will show my secret.

My subtle imperfection will complicate the lives of everyone who loves me.

Shifting perspectives . . .

Kate : Red. Multi-angled.

I had no premonition about Amy.

All my insights are retrospective, as I burrow my way through the folded structures of my brain in search of answers – hunting for clues I might have overlooked, actions which might have made a difference. Medical experts in the field don't apportion blame but however much I'm told it's not my fault, a nagging guilt remains. Because I know I'm selfish. I'm obsessed with my career. I haven't shelved the theatre, despite everything that's happened. In many ways, motherhood was just another role for me.

I'd be reluctant to read a review of that particular performance.

My pregnancy was uneventful. No hint of what lay ahead. The only time I remember feeling sick was prior to the actual diagnosis. That's what sent me to the doctor in the first place. I felt awful. I could hardly lift my head from the pillow. I crawled out to the car and drove off in search of antibiotics. I thought with longing of the days of housecalls. I drooped in the waiting room for over half an hour. I don't know why I ever bother to make an appointment with the fucking doctor. I don't think he's ever seen me on schedule. One day when I was there with Amy, she'd virtually demolished the surgery by the time he saw me. The other patients looked stunned as they watched the drama unfold.

I'd always liked being centre stage – until Amy became my co-star.

The doctor said I had a viral infection. That meant he hadn't a clue what was wrong with me. He didn't prescribe an antibiotic so I haven't got a scapegoat to parade before the jury. He told me to go home and stay in bed. But he took a blood sample and a urine specimen. As a precaution . . .

The sister phoned that afternoon to say he wanted to speak to me about the results.

'Jesus,' I said to Michael. 'It must be bad news. I've never been summoned to the surgery before. Maybe it's cancer. God almighty, I've got fucking cancer. What if I die before the festival?'

Michael had come home that afternoon to minister to his ailing spouse. He took me to the doctor because I felt too shit to drive. He was sitting beside me when the doctor told me I was pregnant.

'Pregnant?' we howled in unison. Like the chorus in a Greek tragedy. We were totally pissed off. It meant I'd be six months pregnant for the festival. It stuffed everything up. We were halfway through workshopping our planned performance. Prof Rankin had launched the country's first actors' centre at the Civic in Johannesburg, based on similar centres he'd worked at in New York and London. It provided both start-up training and mid-career direction so was an ideal place to rendezvous with other actors.

Our piece was called *Five Women*. Different age groups. Different skin tones. My pregnancy meant we had to rework the script to accommodate my swelling belly. It proved a brilliant slice of fortune. We included the theme of the future – a debate on the prospects for a baby born into a rapidly transforming country. It lifted the whole piece beyond the realm of the commonplace. We won the award for best original script that year.

Right from the start, I used Amy to further my career.

Because it was proving so useful, we decided to be delighted about my unexpected pregnancy – although it probably spelled financial ruin. We always faced financial ruin so we thought it wouldn't make much difference.

'You can carry on acting,' said Michael, with his usual blithe assurance. 'We'll get it a backpack and take it everywhere we go. Tom and Sheila hitched around Vietnam with theirs. Ours can be a theatre baby. It won't make any difference. It can't cost much to feed a baby. Some women breastfeed for years. You can be an earth mother – I'll buy you a blanket from the Transkei. It can sleep backstage and absorb the theatre vibe. It'll probably be a hit on Broadway before it gets to playschool.'

So we bought champagne and asked everyone to come to the party. We even asked Claire and Tony – it was a family occasion, after all. My mother was already shopping for the nursery. Tony arrived before Claire, which was unusual. He seldom ventured across the street in front of her – I've never met a more cautious man. We noticed he was different straight away. He walked across the room unsteadily and his speech was slurred when Michael handed him a Scotch. He stood in the middle of the room, swaying slightly and making random conversation. It was out of character.

'Jesus, Kate,' said Michael, under his breath, as we watched from the sidelines. 'I think he's pissed. Maybe the guy's normal after all. They probably both drink and screw like rabbits. We don't really know anything about their lives beyond your mother's Sunday roast.' We seldom felt the urge to socialise with Claire and Tony. We had nothing in common.

At that stage . . .

Claire pushed the buzzer almost ten minutes later. 'Is Tony there?' she asked. 'He said he'd wait for me outside – his car's here but I can't find him anywhere.' I told her to come upstairs and I saw her stiffen when she saw him in the middle of the room. She went straight to him and put his drink on the piano. 'We have to go,' she told me, brusque as ever.

'For God's sake, Claire,' I protested. 'You can't go storming off into the night because the poor bugger's had a few drinks. He's supposed to have a few drinks. It's a celebration! Calm down and have a drink yourself. You have to stay until Dad toasts his pending grandchild. Mom says he's been rehearsing his speech all day. I'm delighted Tony's got a bit drunk for the occasion . . .'

'He's not drunk,' she told me. 'His insulin must be wrong. I've got to get him to a doctor . . .'

Michael and I looked at each other ruefully after we'd helped her put him in the car. We knew Tony was diabetic but we'd never given it a moment's thought. Diabetes was just a word to us.

We had yet to learn that a single word changes everything about your life.

*

Every detail of the day Amy was born is engraved on my mind. An indelible tattoo.

I played the leading role in a miracle.

We loved my pregnant belly. It became our mutual belly as she grew inside me. I lay on the bed like a great, beached whale. We marvelled at my huge extension, at the tautness of my skin with its endless capacity to stretch and hold its secret cargo. I guided Michael's hands so he could feel her moving. We knew she was a girl. We asked them to tell us the sex after the scan. We couldn't wait – I've as little aptitude for patience as for mathematical equations. I could have learned a lot from Claire in both those fields.

I only believed in Amy after my first scan. I was determined not to be pregnant. I thought the symptoms might disappear if I prayed hard enough. A diagnosis can be faulty. I held my breath as I felt the tube sliding up.

And then I saw her on the screen . . .

A tiny capsule of life – like a jelly bean. That's what we called her while I was pregnant. 'What's the news from Jelly Bean today?' Michael asked when he came home. We were

84

forced to believe in her existence because we could hear her heartbeat when we watched the screen that day. We were dazzled to find proof of such a tiny organ – a faint but steady pulse.

We'd made a brand new person.

I asked them to print a copy of her image on the screen. I stuck it on the fridge with a magnet and said hello each time I passed. I added an update from the major scan at twenty weeks – it confirmed a miracle in progress. We both felt excited when I made the appointment. I bought a new dress for the occasion.

'But you're just going to take it off!' protested Michael. He had other plans for how to celebrate the growth spurt of our special bean. 'Let's take her out to dinner. We'll buy expensive wine and let it filter into her bloodstream – give her an early taste of the good things life has to offer.' But I bought the dress anyway. I took it off and watched with trepidation as they applied strategic jelly and attached electrodes to the vital spots. We were electrified to see her image on the screen.

A real baby! Floating in fluid. Moving her arms and legs. It explained all the sensations I'd been feeling. We could see her profile – our first real insight into what she looked like. She popped a tiny thumb into her mouth. We watched her suck for nearly twenty minutes while they measured and did their calculations. They said she was perfect. We felt like giving her a round of applause! We took her out to dinner at the Westcliff to celebrate her commendable statistics. We'd admired the panoramic view of our green city from the balcony when Claire got married – we thought our little stranger should become familiar with the world that was waiting to receive her.

We counted down the days till we could meet her.

My first contraction came at four sixteen that morning. I noted the exact time on the face of my bedside clock. A sharp clench of muscles jolted me awake. At first I dismissed it as another foetal workout session. It felt as if she was doing inter-uterine aerobics as her arrival drew closer. Then the pain came again. And again. My eyes were wide open now. I went to the loo. I padded through and made a cup of tea. I sat down on the sofa to drink it and watched as dawn filtered through the curtains. They need a wash, I thought. I'd never washed my curtains though they'd been hanging there since we moved in. Nearly ten years ago, I thought, inconsequentially.

But I couldn't find a topic to distract me. I focused on the regularity of the pains. It was time for Michael to join the vigil.

'Jesus, Kate!' he said instantly alert, leaping out of bed. Groping for his trousers. 'Let's go! Is everything ready? Where's your bag? Are you going in your nightie?'

'Relax!' I told him, with impressive calm. 'We don't want to get there too early. They'll send us home. Let's have a drink before we leave.'

'A drink?' he asked in disbelief. 'For Christ's sake, you can't have a drink. The sun's just coming up. They'll be serving morning tea at the hospital. They won't admit you if you pitch up pissed. I'll have to deliver her myself in the fucking corridor!'

But we had a drink. We had champagne and orange juice in tall, long-stemmed glasses. We'd bought them specially to welcome our new trio home – to declare ourselves officially a family. Michael popped the cork and proposed a toast to whoever was about to join us. He sat down at the piano and said he'd play a new tune with each contraction. When his medley picked up sufficient speed, we collected my pre-packed suitcase and hurried to the car. We were excited! I waved at the early morning people at the robots. Michael wound down his window and told the couple in the car that drew up beside us. They laughed and clapped and wished us well.

I felt like a celebrity!

It got less exciting. More painful. Michael sat beside me. Rubbed my back. Wiped my sweaty face with a cool damp cloth. Held the glass while I drank a sip of water. I was so thirsty. I braced myself as the pain arched through my body. I felt the cold stethoscope as they listened for the heartbeat and monitored the journey.

'How much longer?' I thought I couldn't bear it.

And then, suddenly, I was aware of sliding. Lubrication. A swift rush and the pain was over . . .

'You've got a lovely daughter,' smiled the doctor, as he placed her in my arms.

A miracle.

✳

I'm a passionate person. I'm seldom neutral about any topic so intensity isn't unfamiliar – but I still felt overwhelmed when I held our little daughter. Her smell. The soft down on her head. Her compact body, perfect in its smallest details.

I wonder if it's true to say I love her more than anything

I've encountered in my world.

Until Amy's arrival, my feelings for Michael dwarfed every other relationship. We still share common goals and passions. We lose our tempers. Hurl accusations. Use careless words that bleed and damage all we have together – but we always reconcile. And sex can heal the deepest wounds . . .

I'm different from my friends. They've all had several sexual partners. More than several. One night stands. New relationships. It wasn't like that for me. It's not that I'm a disciple of monogamy – I'm not morally superior to my friends who sleep around. I was sexually active, years before most of them got started. But I've never needed anyone but Michael. He turns me on. I sometimes feel I might explode with pleasure when our bodies lock together, when the final jigsaw piece slots into place. I've never had another lover.

I don't know if it's the same for him. We're so distant now. We're poles apart, even when the sex is good. Our hot bodies contradict our icy feelings.

It wasn't like that when Amy was born. Michael wasn't just my baby's father – he was my closest friend. He'd be Amy's most formidable rival in a contest gauging who I loved the most. Perhaps the judge would invalidate the whole procedure – on the grounds that the contestants aren't true rivals. They're not in competition with each other.

I can't compare the love I feel for Amy with any other love I've ever felt.

She's mine. A tiny dependant. Locked to my breast with toothless gums and clutching fingers. We were delighted with her toes and fingers, each fitted with a perfect crescent nail. We smiled at her wrinkled face and baby noises as she drank and settled down to sleep. We thought we were bloody marvellous. That's why we called her Amy.

'We've found our forte,' Michael told me. 'We owe it to the world to produce an entire alphabet of babies. This one can be Amy. We'll follow up with Bill and Catherine. Then we'll have David. We'll alternate sexes. We'll have one every year!'

It seemed a good idea. Everyone remarked on the beauty of our baby as she grew into her skin and lost her wrinkles. A porcelain girl. I could hardly believe she was mine. The gods had obviously made a decision to compensate the ugly sister for the plain face she'd grown up with. They gave us the most beautiful baby on the planet.

Amy looks just like Claire.

Michael doted on her from the outset. He was as involved as I was. He didn't go off to work from nine to five like other fathers. He was around to help at bath time, to walk her round and pat her back when she screamed her head off. She slept in a carrycot beside our bed in those early months. When she cried, he got up and changed her nappy. He latched her on my sleepy breast – I'd feed her, listen for a burp that might be causing her discomfort. I'd snuggle down and let her fall asleep between us.

It wasn't long before we rotated the feeding shift. I weaned her early. For convenience. I was always focused on what would be the easiest for me. The doctors have assured me that can't be what caused it – but they don't know everything. Maybe it all adds up to some kind of retribution – we made no effort at all to adapt our lives to Amy. We expected her to fit in with what we did. She attended as many rehearsals as the rest of the cast. She had no routine at all. She was passed around backstage. Someone fed her. Someone changed her nappy if she cried. Usually.

Sometimes she was completely overlooked.

I came off stage one night, after the final curtain, flushed with applause for my performance. Aglow with success. The dressing room door was closed but I could hear her crying. I found her standing in her campcot, tears streaming down her face. Alone. In a dark room. I picked her up and covered her with kisses. I knew she could have been crying for as long as I'd been on stage. Over an hour . . .

There has to be an element of retribution in all that's happened since.

But despite my daily guilt trip, we didn't waste that patch of stress-free time allotted by the gods who oversee these matters. We adored our baby. She was our princess. Our pineapple pie. Our chocolate doughnut. She crawled around, exploring. Tottered to her feet and started walking. She talked on schedule. Michael made up tunes on the piano and sang her special songs. Written just for her. He whirled her round and got her dancing. He took her with him to Pretoria where he was rehearsing – he'd been cast as *The Curious Cat. The Rum Tum Tugger.* A local impresario had bought the rights to stage the Broadway hit.

Maybe that's what started Amy's cat fixation. I made us ears and whiskers and a tail to swish behind. Her father sat at the piano, strumming the familiar tune.

The Rum Tum Tugger is a Curious Cat.

Amy and I circled behind him, clapping our paws in time to the music, our tails held high. We developed a ritual.

When Michael finished a verse, he'd spin round on the piano stool and bellow, 'Who's Rum Tum Tugger?' Amy and I would scream, 'A silly bugger!' and shriek with laughter. Michael threw his bewhiskered princess in the air and spun her round and round.

I'll never be as happy as I was then.

It's ironic that of all the cats on the menu, Michael got the part of Rum Tum Tugger. He brought the house down with his take-off of Mick Jagger – a leather-coated feline. Sinuous, suggestive hips. Tight buns. A mane of wild hair, flouncing and strutting provocatively among the other dancers. Belting out the lyrics . . .

Yes the Rum Tum Tugger is a Curious Cat –
And it isn't any use for you to doubt it:
For he will do
As he do do
And there's no doing anything about it!

He could have been describing Amy.

✻

Amy's problems were triggered by her MMR vaccination.

Measles, mumps, rubella – I'd have all three, in plague proportions, in exchange for what I got instead.

Claire says I'm wrong. She downloads all the latest research refuting the connection. She recently showed me a report from the Medical Research Council in the UK which indicates the lack of convincing scientific support for the theory. While it confirms the increasing prevalence of the disorder, it cites large-scale studies to suggest that vaccination doesn't result in earlier exposure of the symptoms. It points out that the incidence is the same in children who weren't immunised. I suppose it's the same as blaming teenage suicide on Roaccutane – the miracle acne drug. When the parents of the dead protest, the pharmaceutical giant responds with a press release that teenagers are prone to depression and suicide. And it's the same with vaccinations. Instead, the report points fingers at gene malfunction. Subtle neonatal changes in the structure of the brain stem. They conclude that it's unlikely – even impossible – to link it to the MMR.

But they weren't there. Those doctors didn't have to watch our princess turn into a stranger. Amy was just like all the other little girls till I gave her that injection. It was like a fairy story, back to front. We all know about frogs and Prince Charming. Metamorphosis. That's an uplifting experience in biology – an unfurling of potential. But for us, the movie was rewinding. Going backwards. Our butterfly didn't open her wings and soar into the sky. She folded them around her and crept back into her cocoon.

There was nothing we could do to stop her.

Amy was nearly eighteen months before she had her vaccination. I was such a slapdash mother, I didn't get around to doing it on schedule. My mother was constantly reminding me.

'You don't want her to get measles,' she warned me. 'They can be very sick with measles. Run a high temperature. And the rash frightens them . . .'

I blamed her for this advice, in retrospect. I blamed everybody. I was desperate to find someone who was guilty.

Guiltier than me.

I remember the day I took her to the doctor for her routine jab. She was still talking then – jabbering away as I buckled her shoes and tied her hair in a jaunty ponytail on top of her head. She looked so cute. It's one of the photos I have in my file of memories. My before and after box.

'We're going to see the doctor!' I told her. 'He'll give you a little prick – but it won't hurt because I'll be with you.'

'See the doctor!' chirped my little parrot. 'Little prick.'

That was a good description of the doctor – but my judgement is probably clouded through association. He was the one who gave her the injection – and his was the first medical opinion I heard when I dared to raise the word Tony and Claire suggested. I hated them all. I would have thrown the Angel Gabriel into the deepest, darkest dungeon if he'd been the one to hold the needle, if he'd planted the suggestion in my mind.

The injection gave Amy a high fever. We were up all night with her. She felt like a furnace. Michael held her on his lap while I wiped her down with a cool, damp cloth – as our well-thumbed baby manual suggested. I phoned the doctor early next morning but he said it was a normal reaction. Nothing to worry about. And when I'm thinking clearly, I accept that this is probably true. I'm not a doctor. I know fuck all about the workings of the human body. Everyone in our circle had her baby vaccinated. Other babies had a feverish response.

The mothers at the clinic were reassuring.

'Jenny was just like that,' one told me, patting my arm, bouncing the Jenny in question on her lap. A pigtailed, chatty

Jenny. Unpacking the toybox. Giggling, pointing to the mobile. But Amy was different. Different from Jenny at the clinic. Different from the children of our friends and neighbours. And different from both her parents.

Michael and I both thrive on human contact. Our livelihood depends on feedback from the audience. If we don't make that connection, we're history. It's much harder to make that connection if you don't share a common language. Like watching an opera without subtitles. You have to guess what they're trying to say. Amy said less and less as she got older. We didn't know what she wanted. She wouldn't let anyone cross her boundaries. We couldn't find a way to reach her.

A chain of thought passed through my mind one night as I lay in bed after a particularly dreadful day – some days were worse than others. Maybe it was all a dream. Maybe we'd been cast in a stage adaptation of *The Midwich Cuckoos*. I remember thinking the book would make an effective play when I read it at Drama School. I was looking for a suitable text to use in the scriptwriting course. We had to write a screenplay from a novel. Wyndham's story caught my imagination – alien children planted in the homes of the unsuspecting population of a small English village. Effective on the stage if you cast it well – baffled, uncomprehending parents struggling to come to terms with their changeling children.

It felt like we were living through that plot – trying to establish contact with a little person who was fundamentally different. Intrinsically strange. Our princess had climbed up to the top of her ivory tower. The doctors said she wasn't deaf but that didn't mean that she could hear us.

We felt completely helpless. We had to stand on the sidelines while Amy evolved into an alien. We didn't have a whistle we could blow to change the course her life was taking.

*

Michael was first to feel a sense of unease. Even that makes me guilty. I should have been the one to notice. But I had regular work at the time. I'd signed a six month contract to appear in a local series aimed to heighten AIDS awareness in the community. I played a housewife learning to adapt to her maid's positive diagnosis, preparing to cope with the hazards ahead.

I was too busy to notice the hazards developing at home.

'Has Amy got her full quota of teeth?' Michael asked me. 'She's been off colour for a while. I'm going to have to jack up my repertoire – I can't seem to get a smile out of her these days. She won't even look at me, let alone sing along and trip the light fantastic. She's so quiet – she's shelved our early morning chat show. I'm worried.'

'It probably is a tooth,' I told him. 'I'll put some of the stuff on her gums tonight. She'll be fine.'

But she wasn't fine. Next day was Saturday and I bunged the washing that had been building up all week into the machine. Then I went to shower and wash my hair. When I was ready to leave, I couldn't find Amy anywhere.

'Amy!' I yelled. 'Mummy's ready! Where are you hiding?'

She didn't answer. I looked in the bedroom by the toybox. Everything was in order. She was very tidy for a little girl. I thought she might be watching a cartoon in the

TV room. Empty. I found her in the kitchen where I'd left her over forty minutes ago. She was staring at the washing. Going round and round. Water and soapflakes and a mass of tangled clothes. It had already reached the spin cycle — revolving in endless circles.

'Amy!' I called again. 'Come on darling. I'm ready now.'

But she didn't turn around. She didn't seem to hear me. She was transfixed. Not fidgeting or pointing or trying to open the machine. She just watched it spin. As if hypnotised . . .

It was almost eerie. It scared me. I mentioned the incident to Michael that evening.

'Really?' he asked, looking anxious. 'I had a similar thing last week. I looked everywhere for her. I found her in a corner of our bedroom. Just rocking. Backwards and forwards. Over and over. I tried to make her laugh but she wouldn't look at me. I'm struggling to get her to look at me, now I think about it. She's very withdrawn. Almost aloof. Do you think she can hear us? Maybe we should have her ears tested. Perhaps she's deaf.'

We were anxious. Naturally, I asked my mother. And naturally she said Amy was perfect. As perfect as Claire and I had always been. Amy reminded her of Claire as a baby – and not just because they look alike.

'Claire was also a quiet little girl,' she told me. 'She'd sit for hours in her playpen, just looking at pools of sunlight slanting through the curtains. She was such a good baby – broke us in gently. I think you always worry more about your first child because you don't know what to expect. You don't know what's normal because you've nothing to compare it with. You were so different. Much more adventurous. I'm sure it's because Dad and I were both more relaxed the second time around.'

I wasn't reassured.

I was glad Amy looked like Claire – but that's as far as I wanted the resemblance to go. I was happy to restrict my exposure to my sister to the occasional Sunday lunch with my parents to dilute her.

I didn't want her in the cot beside our bed.

✳

I resented Claire's relationship with Amy.

Not because I wanted a similar relationship. I don't think Claire and I view a relationship in the same light. For me, it implies a two-way connection. Like an electrical circuit. If you have a relationship with a person, there must be a current that flows between you. I'm not talking about sex – that's in a different category. It has a special niche all on its own. I'm thinking of relationships without a sexual basis.

Take my relationship with my mother. We sometimes despair of each other but we definitely have a relationship. We'll share a joke. Phone each other if we're sad. Or if we're happy. We talk about a topic, even if we disagree. Claire and Amy don't have a link like that. Nor do Claire and Tony.

It's hard to put your finger on what connects Claire to other people. It sounds contradictory but I think the common factor in all her relationships is distance. Whether it's the safety of cyberspace or some local, individual barrier. She'll freeze out anyone who tries to cross her boundaries. Claire's very territorial. Like a cat. Maybe that appeals to Amy, with her feline fetish. No one ever really knows what

Claire is thinking. Tony's a mystery too. He never offers an opinion on anything not work-related. And I haven't a clue what goes on in Amy's mind. All three of them operate on closed circuits. Dependent on each other but essentially independent. It's too complicated for me.

I'm on the outside of that trio. I don't know the magic password, despite my blood connections. I'm being denied a birthright. Amy's my daughter. I love her. It's wrong that our circuits aren't connected. I want to pick up my child and hold her little body, warm and tight and safe against me. I want her to stop crying. I want to cover her with kisses. Make her better.

But she stiffens when I do that. Turns her head away. Not only from me. From Michael too. From everyone. The textbooks say she's tactile defensive. Claire's the same so she's content to leave Amy alone in her corner. Or under her bed. It suits both of them.

But it doesn't suit me. I'm jealous that it suits them both so well.

As always, I have only myself to blame. I introduced Claire into the Amy equation. She didn't volunteer or elbow her way into the picture – that's not Claire's style. I needed a babysitter. For my own convenience. So that I didn't have to opt out of the play I was working on. I had a demanding schedule of rehearsals. Amy's behaviour had deteriorated to such an extent that I couldn't take her with me any more.

'All children go through a stage where they seem impossible,' my mother told me, in comfort mode as usual. I kept repeating that mantra to myself when Amy screamed and kicked and bit her way through an afternoon. I often screamed back. I was sorely tempted to kick and bite as well. I did shake her sometimes. I took her by her fragile shoulders and shook her like a rag doll. Like a fluttering bird. It didn't stop her. She got more frenzied. I forced myself to let her go. Walk away. I leaned my head against the wall. Gutted. And guilty. I thought I'd drown in guilt when I registered how small and frail my target was, sobbing in a pile of tangled limbs.

Amy's beautiful. Somehow it made everything worse. I was shocked that someone so small and beautiful could make me lose my temper. Feel so violent. I was used to war with Michael but he's an enemy worthy of my steel. He can stand up for himself.

Amy couldn't stand up for herself. She'd retrogressed. She was back in nappies. Not like her peers. I thought I'd done something wrong. Failed some mother-instinct test. I was reluctant to leave her at the homes of friends with all their potty-trained children playing constructive, educational games together. I couldn't predict how Amy would behave. My friends stopped offering to help. They sometimes looked as if they'd survived a tornado when I went to pick her up. I knew what they'd been through. On other days, she went to the opposite extreme. That was also disconcerting. She was like the little girl in the poem – when she was good she was very, very good . . .

'She's been an absolute angel,' said Elaine. 'You're so lucky. Stevie's still hurtling round the house like Michael Schumacher – Amy's been no trouble at all. I hardly knew she was here. Stevie wanted her to join his Grand Prix circuit but she wasn't interested. But she liked one of the cars. She's been sitting spinning its wheels ever since Stevie gave it to her. She's got an amazing attention span for such a little girl. Stevie gets bored after five minutes and I have to find some new form of entertainment. You're lucky she's so independent,' she repeated.

But I didn't feel lucky as I made my way home with Amy silent in the seat behind me. Not telling me what she'd been up to. Not eager for my approval. She hardly seemed aware of my existence. She wasn't performing the role I wanted my daughter to play. And I wouldn't get an Oscar for my performance as her mother. It wasn't enough that Amy was beautiful. A child star has to learn her words as well. Amy wasn't using the script I wanted her to follow. She said less and less as she got older.

'Nonsense!' said my mother when I told her I was worried. 'She talks perfectly well when she wants to. And her memory is amazing. The last time she was here, she recited that little rhyme you use as a voice exercise sometimes.'

'What little rhyme?' I asked her blankly.

'You know the one. I've often heard you say it when you're trying to loosen up before a performance. It's quite complicated. I can't say it, even though I've heard you use it several times. Something about sitting in silence. And a short sharp shock. She remembered the whole thing, word for word.'

I felt cold. I knew the verse she meant. *The Mikado*. It's effective as a warm-up because it requires quite a bit of vocal dexterity – but it makes no sense out of context. It would be nonsense to a toddler. Very complicated nonsense. My mind ran through the words . . .

To sit in sudden silence in a dull dark dock
Awaiting the sensation of a short sharp shock

In a penitential prison with a life long lock
And a cheap and chippy chopper on a big black block.

The verse wasn't the only thing that didn't make sense. Why could my little girl recite complicated nonsense when she couldn't tell me the name of the everyday items I showed her in the kitchen?

'Don't worry darling,' said my mother. Inevitably. As always. I could see I was going to have to shoot my mother before long. 'Claire was just the same. She used to recite grocery lists. Any list she could find. It worried me dreadfully at the time but she grew out of it. Amy will too. It's a just a stage.'

Just a stage. That's what they all said. Every conversation about Amy seemed to end with that refrain. It made me unwilling to leave Amy with anyone other than my mother. I never knew what stage Amy might decide to go through at any given time. I was embarrassed. Ashamed of my picture-book daughter. I didn't know where to leave her if my parents were away, if Michael was also busy with rehearsals. I should have cancelled what I was doing and looked after her myself. But I liked what I was doing. Sacrifice is not my forte.

So I asked Claire and Tony to babysit. I exploited them. It didn't matter what they thought of Amy. Their opinion was irrelevant to me. And besides, they never gave me an opinion. I used them more and more. They didn't pass a comment when I arrived to pick her up. They never told me how she'd behaved.

I didn't ask. I didn't want to know.

The afternoons Amy spent with Claire and Tony gave

me respite from Amy. She drained my emotional resources. I was exhausted. Michael was touring with *Fantasticks*. I was desperate for a break so I took advantage of the fact that they were always willing to have her. They seemed to have no social commitments. They worked from nine to five during the week. And at the weekend, they looked after Amy. It developed into a pattern. It was wonderful not to have to listen to any more advice on how to rectify Amy's multiple failings.

I valued their silence on the progress she wasn't making.

✳

It's ironic that it was Claire and Tony who were the ones who forced me to admit the truth about Amy.

I can recall the afternoon – down to the finest detail. The date. The weather. Even what we were wearing. I remember a Drew Barrymore movie – *Riding in Cars with Boys*. Two of her lines made an impact. Lingered where I filed them in my bank of Amy memories. She said your whole life boils down to a couple of days when everything changes. And she wondered if she loved her son just because she had to. Both those thoughts have crossed my mind.

The day Claire abandoned her no-comment routine will always be of the utmost significance for me.

She didn't complain about Amy's behaviour. She didn't say she'd thrown a brick through the computer screen. It wasn't some ordinary demolition issue. I don't think Claire would have mentioned that. Tony would just have bought a new one on the quiet. They never made me feel guilty about leaving Amy with them. Claire only broke her silence because she thought I'd be delighted. She thought I'd be as excited as they were.

Amy hadn't done anything dreadful. She'd been remarkable.

I rang the buzzer early that evening. A faint chill. Winter just around the corner. Claire let me in. Tony was behind her, holding Amy by the hand. Her hair was in plaits. Blue ribbons. She looked like Alice in Wonderland.

'You'll never believe what Amy did this afternoon!' said Claire. Immediately. She didn't even say hello.

My heart sank like a stone.

'Tell me the worst,' I said bravely. 'Is it going to cost a fortune? Is one of you maimed for life?'

'No! No!' Claire assured me. 'It's wonderful! She's the most amazing child. You won't believe it! I'd never have believed it myself, if I hadn't watched her with my own eyes. Tony still can't believe it!'

'What did she do?' I asked, hope welling up inside me, like an oil strike in Texas. I couldn't imagine what was coming. Maybe she'd suddenly started to speak in sentences. Even a paragraph?

'What did she do? Tell me!' I begged, bursting with impatience.

'I came in to clear up and get her ready to go,' Claire told me, her face lit up like a candle. It was unusual to hear her sound excited. 'Amy was lying on the floor, scribbling. She looked really awkward. Her face was about an inch from the paper. She was drawing very quickly – it looked like a hotchpotch of lines. A jumble. Her pencil was moving all the time – she hardly lifted it off the paper. And then she stopped. I thought it was just another page of scribbling

so I didn't even look at it. I swept it up with everything else
– that's why the page is so crumpled. But it caught my eye
when I went throw it in the dustbin. I can't believe what
she's done. Just look at this!'

She handed me a sheet of crumpled paper, smoothed
out and open.

Claire's Siamese cat looked back at me. Anna. I always
thought it an inappropriate name for a Siamese but Claire
never seems aware of incongruity. Association is the guiding
principle for her. She chose the name because of *The King
and I*. Anna and the King of Siam. Claire's cat could certainly
have been the consort of kings. She was an aristocrat. Sleek.
Elegant. Patrician. A feline version of my sister.

Amy had captured all those qualities on her crumpled
sheet of paper. She hadn't used a rigid outline. There were
light flowing lines. A variety of marks and smudges. But
she somehow conveyed the texture of Anna's fur. Densely
packed strokes where her coat was darker. Loose open
stokes – a suggestion of a lighter tone. Anna's a complicated
cat. Subtle. Amy's drawing had perspective – an overall
sense of proportion. It captured the essence of the cat,
although it lacked the finer details.

It was remarkable. Too sophisticated for a child of
Amy's age. For a child of any age. Even for an adult. I
couldn't have reproduced it.

It made me feel sick. I crumpled it in my hand and thrust
it blindly into the pocket of my coat. Claire and Tony
looked bewildered as I took Amy's hand and pulled her
down the stairs behind me.

My hands were shaking. I could hardly start the car.

Because I knew then that I'd have to face it. I could explain

away the tantrums. The words she failed to speak. Her
remoteness. Her peculiar play. But I couldn't explain this.
The just-a-stage refrain was rendered useless in the context
of that drawing.

There was something seriously wrong with Amy.

Amy : Circular. Colour-coded.

I live in a kaleidoscope. I'm trapped. Profoundly alone – although I don't feel lonely. My world has no boundaries. Past and present overlap. Replays. Rewinding. Nothing makes sense. Sights and sounds. Shapes. Taste. Colour. An incoherent jumble of sensation. Everything changes. It's as if I've been awakened by a stranger in the middle of a dark and moonless night. I don't understand his reasons. He thrusts me in a suitcase. I hear the key turn. He drives me along unfamiliar roads towards a foreign airport.

I can't escape from the suitcase. A cacophony of sounds crowd in around me, invading the small space I've been allotted. It's overwhelming. The hum of traffic. Brakes squealing. Birdsong. Voices. Loud and soft. Near or far. I can't understand the words they use. They relate to nothing that's familiar to me.

I'm terrified. I kick and flail my arms, desperate for freedom.

He opens the suitcase when we reach the airport. The daylight's blinding. Myriad colours. Red. Blue. Green and orange. Neon lights flashing. On and off. It hurts my eyes. I'm dazzled. I don't recognise anything or anyone. They speak a foreign language. I can't understand their instructions. There are crowds of people – all going somewhere. Except me. I have no idea of my destination, of what I'm expected to do. I can't anticipate what's going to happen next. I try to pull the threads together but they form an incoherent picture. A blurred impression. The outline is unfamiliar.

I scream because I'm frightened. The world makes no sense to me.

I learn some words through repetition. They become familiar so they trigger a reaction. I yearn for things I can predict. Sameness and security are synonyms for me. I know the faces I see often – but the words that name them change. It's confusing. I can't work out the pattern. Kate. Michael. Darling. Mummy and daddy. Princess. Claire and Tony. Which is which? Who do they mean? Me. You. Him and her. Mine and yours. Amy's?

I can't decode the reference system.

But I feel more secure when they're with me. I know their voices. The shape of their bodies. Their laps. The bed. The layout of the house we live in. I still get frightened, even when it seems familiar. Because they assault me. Too many

107

kisses. Moist, pursed lips against my skin. Like an octopus. They hold me too tightly. Sweep me off the floor and spin me round until I'm dizzy. I feel like I've been high-jacked. And they change. Sometimes they laugh. Or sing. Or shout. Open mouths with teeth and tongues. Like sharks . . .

I'm terrified.

They won't leave me alone. They change my clothes. Bath me. Cut my hair. My skin rebels when I'm exposed to different textures. Too rough. My pores cry out in protest. A plague of ants. And then too soft. As sinister as silk, smooth and sliding. I find the water overwhelming. Its wetness. Too hot. Or too cold. I'm drowning. I feel the cold metal of the scissors on my cheek. Reflections dance before me in the glass. I'm bewildered by the clouds and sunshine. Light and dark. Day and night.

I'm living through a nightmare.

But sometimes I escape. Find a place to hide. Shut them out. I wedge myself into a corner. I feel the solid wall against my back. The floor is stable. I rock. Backwards and forwards. I flap my hands and twirl a strand of hair between my fingers. I walk on tiptoe through my dreamscape. No one's watching as I spin the wheels. Round and round. Endless turning . . .

It calms me. It restores order.

I wish I could be caught in a time warp in those quiet moments. I crave a structured world. Frozen forever. Captured by a camera. Safe and far away. Sealed inside a capsule, in the galaxy's most distant reaches, the dark spaces of the universe.

Silent. Uniform. Predictable.

Alone on my planet.

Tony : Sepia. Background blended.

Claire and I had no expectations of Amy. That's why she hasn't been a trauma for us. She doesn't bruise and batter our emotions. We know she's complicated but we accept her as she is.

She's just Amy.

It's easier for us – we're not her parents. We didn't start off with a pocketful of dreams of all she might achieve. Perhaps Kate and Michael still hope there's another little girl inside. A happier girl than Amy. Someone more like them. They're so passionate about everything – particularly about Amy. I get the feeling, as time passes, that they love her more than they love each other. They're desperate to find a key to turn and set her free. It's hard to abandon a dream — or so they say.

I've never been a dreamer.

Claire and I had no children in our future plans. We considered the future only in terms of retirement annuities and financial planning. Amy wasn't a factor we'd keyed into our futures' portfolio. We didn't anticipate that she'd become the focal point of every conversation we hold outside the office. Even in the office. At unguarded moments, I find her there — in my thoughts, in my weekend prospects. We're more immersed in Amy than in the AIDS project that introduced us at the outset.

It's strange. She's only a niece — that's not a significant bond for anyone. Especially when sisterhood is as faint a connection as it is for Claire. Our contact with Kate was minimal until after Amy's second birthday — on the surface anyway. Claire seldom mentioned her sister but she seemed an undercover disciple. Her scrapbook of Kate's theatrical career is comprehensive. Programmes. Reviews. Photographs. Nothing's missing. Kate should use that scrapbook as a CV — she's unlikely to have kept a systematic record of her own.

I also like to watch Kate on stage — though I have to draw the line on occasion. I can't get past the title sometimes. I'd feel like a voyeur if I joined the audience. All that raw emotion. Feelings I've never had myself. It would be like watching through a keyhole. Spying on something private. Intimacy repels me. My mother's blueprint must be embedded in my psyche — I'm intrinsically conservative.

Amy's the most offbeat aspect of my life.

The prospect of fatherhood is never one I've entertained

– and not only because of my diabetes. I have no idea what to say to a child – even when I was a child myself. I avoid children. It's harder than talking to Kate and Michael – and those conversations are always stilted. But I don't have to hold a conversation with Amy. Even when she talks to me, it's not a two-way stream. She doesn't expect a response. She has no interest in how I feel about a situation. She doesn't care if I'm pleased with her or not.

She's tailor-made for Claire and me.

※

I can't claim that Amy slotted into our lives like the missing piece of a jigsaw puzzle. I don't think either of us will ever forget the first afternoon she spent with us in charge. It was a nightmare. We could have used the services of a trauma counsellor – I think it would have been less stressful to be hijacked at gunpoint.

We were both aghast after Kate phoned that Friday evening. Claire's face is not expressive – I'm seldom certain what she's thinking, even after all our years together. But I could see there was a problem when she ended the conversation – she looked almost dumbfounded.

'That was Kate,' she told me – to my surprise. Kate never phoned. I assumed it was related to their parents. Claire's father had won a staff incentive – we'd waved them farewell at the airport in a flurry of excitement as they headed off on a Caribbean cruise. But Claire shook her head when I asked how the trip was going.

'She wants us to have Amy tomorrow afternoon,' she told me. 'She's got a dress rehearsal and her babysitter's let her down.'

'She wants to leave her here?' I asked in disbelief. 'All afternoon? But what will we do with her?'

We'd always kept our distance from the new addition to the family. Everyone else treated her like the crown jewels. But Claire didn't want to hold her or bounce her on her knee. She never offered to read her a story. Even I paid Amy more attention than Claire did. I couldn't take my eyes off her – she looked so much like Claire. It was as if my wife had shrunk in the wash. It felt strange to see Claire in miniature. Amy was like a toy – but not one I wanted to play with.

We found Amy very irritating. Our hearts sank if Michael's ancient Ford was parked outside Claire's mother's house when we arrived for Sunday lunch. Amy seemed to cry all the time. And so loudly. She was very destructive – Kate and Michael both looked exhausted as they scrambled in her wake. Amy's a very pretty little girl – but her behaviour was erratic. Some afternoons we'd hardly notice she was there – she sat on her cushion in the corner – but most times, she made her presence felt. We were always the first to leave when Amy came to visit Granny. The prospect of an afternoon alone with her was more daunting than a presentation to the board of any corporate giant.

We did a special trip on Saturday morning to prepare for the occasion. Kate said she'd bring a box of toys to keep her busy but we thought we should invest in some back-up resources. Just in case. We bought extra crayons. A colouring book. An omnibus of fairy tales. A large jigsaw. Enough sweets to feed an entire class at nursery school. We hoped to bribe her into silence.

We braced ourselves for a storm of protest when Kate said goodbye and closed the door behind her. But Amy didn't seem to notice she'd gone. She was watching Anna – who ignored her completely. Anna is as unsociable a cat as her owner. She continued washing her paws, oblivious of Amy's concentrated attention.

We felt ill at ease in the unexpected silence. Should we interrupt? Suggest a game? Open the toy-box? Tell a story? Was it too soon to offer a sweet?

We had no idea how to entertain a toddler.

Anna solved the problem. She stretched in her languid fashion and began to move towards a patch of sunshine on the table. Amy immediately tried to stop her – we've since learned that Amy likes everything to stay in one place. She took hold of Anna and tried to put her back on the chair where she'd been sitting. That set the afternoon in motion. In a downward spiral. Anna objected. She wasn't used to interference. She growled and lashed out at Amy's face, claws unsheathed in protest. But Amy didn't drop her. She held her tighter. She didn't seem to notice the scratch marks raked in a jagged line across her face. Ignored Claire when she told her to let the cat go. Anna's protests became more frenzied – I had to pull Amy's arms apart to set her free. Amy was outraged – she unleashed a piercing scream and tried to grab the cat back from me. Anna leapt out of my arms and dislodged a china ashtray which shattered on the tiled floor underneath the table.

It was awful. Five minutes had passed since Amy's arrival. Her face was scratched and bleeding. She sounded as if she was being murdered. I wouldn't have been surprised to see our neighbour. Or the police. There was broken china on the floor and a bristling, spitting feline on the table.

It was a long afternoon

We felt like holocaust survivors when Kate finally closed the door behind them that evening. She was an hour later than she said she'd be. Flustered apologies. They'd had to rerun the scene. Etcetera. Etcetera. We were past listening at that stage. I saw Kate flinch as she registered the conditions in our lounge – our immaculate lounge. Helter-skelter cushions. Half-eaten sweets – our bribery campaign hadn't proved as successful as with local politicians. We'd certainly been tempted to try the other South African solution to problems. Violence . . .

Baby-bashing didn't seem as inexplicable as usual after an afternoon with Amy.

But none of us said anything. Nothing relating to the chaos. We passed a few brittle pleasantries. How's the play coming along? Have you had a lovely time darling?

Thanks so much. Goodbye. Kate sounded like Anne Robinson on BBC. She took the family's weakest link by the hand and headed out into the evening.

We were speechless.

❋

Amy wasn't speechless although she was often silent.

Like Claire and me. The odd couple – with an extension odder than both of us. A triad of impairments. We grew more familiar with that phrase when Amy's diagnosis was confirmed. It seems to sum us up. A man, a woman and a child – it should add up to marriage and a family. I'm sure that's what the priest expected when he spoke to us that day. His words echoed in the almost empty church. For better or for worse. In sickness and in health. Till death us do part. They don't sound incongruous – even though we'll never fit the standard profile.

I'm certain the three of us will be linked forever.

Legally, our marriage is null and void. It's never been consummated. We've never had sex – although we always sleep together. Not in each other's arms. Side by side. Perhaps it doesn't matter in the new millennium. Marriage is a looser term today. Anything goes – same gender, common law wife, test-tube babies – everything's more flexible than when they wrote the Bible. I've never read the Bible. I don't know who chose the words for the marriage service but they've lasted longer than the Beatles. Statistically, the Bible is the world's best-seller. Perhaps it contains an element of truth for every situation.

It's not a reference book Claire uses. She preaches the gospel according to the Oxford. Everything is cut and dried for Claire. Black and white. Claire's oblivious to nuance. The Oxford says a parent is one who has begotten offspring. And a daughter is a female child. Claire knows that neither term applies to us. We aren't a threat to Kate and Michael. Our triad is completely different from theirs.

The Oxford mentions parent-teacher as a subgroup of parents – an organisation consisting of and promoting good relations between teachers and parents. And it says a daughter can be the spiritual or intellectual product of a person. Those definitions contain an element of truth. Perhaps that's our category. Amy's linked to Kate and Michael – and she's also linked to Claire and me. Both triads are impaired. Neither functions effectively alone – but when we combine them, when we act in concert, harmony sometimes seems a goal we can aspire to.

I work with the mathematical definition of harmony – quantities whose reciprocals are in arithmetical progression. Reciprocity. The principle of give and take. Interchange of privileges. It all applies. One should never underestimate the Oxford. It has a lot to say about speech and silence for example. They're inextricably linked, according to the Oxford. Silence is abstinence from speech. And abstinence implies the sacrifice of something pleasurable. But I don't think conversation is a pleasurable activity for Claire or Amy.

Their silence is different from mine. I'm quiet because of shyness. I've always been self-conscious. Anxious. Are my words appropriate? Will they think I'm stupid? That's why I'm a loner. I try to avoid situations which might provoke a negative response from other people. Neither Claire nor Amy is silent for that reason. They're much more self-contained than I am. Speech has no more significance than other sounds for them. They're both visual thinkers – they don't automatically use language as a tool for thinking. Claire's not sensitive to tone like I am. To her, words mean exactly what the Oxford says they mean. I don't think it simplifies her life. It makes everything more complicated. Sarcasm at the office is wasted on Claire. She often misses the point when she hears a joke. I understand the jokes but I seldom have the confidence to laugh. I've never felt part of a group. It's one of my impairments.

But I think all three of us have been born into the right millennium. The computer is as significant in this century as a car was in the last. I read *The Mail & Guardian* as avidly

116

as Claire reads the Oxford. They featured an article recently on the link between technological advances and social phobia. I felt as if I was looking in the mirror.

For many people, every day is a struggle with debilitating social anxiety. Routine actions such as eating or drinking are complicated by an irrational fear of scrutiny. Casual conversation is an ordeal. Social and occupational functioning can eventually become impaired, resulting in a sense of isolation. Social phobia is in a different category to simple shyness and appears to be on the increase. Is technology to blame? ATMs, answering machines and e-mail reduce the need for social contact in the new millennium. The Mayo Clinic has recently completed a study highlighting the potential dangers of a wired world. People become so obsessed with the Internet that real-time relationships fade into insignificance. Today, you can even confide in your therapist on-line – that's big business in the States and Europe.

Our triad is wired to a dangerous degree. A computer is as invaluable to us as a car – or even our daily bread. It's more addictive than tobacco or alcohol. Claire keeps up to date with all the latest theories that relate to Amy. It's like an obsession. She's probably qualified to make a speech or write a textbook. And Amy's been dexterous with a mouse since her first introduction. She likes the repetition. Predictable answers. She plays her favourite games over and over again. Her attention span's remarkable for a child.

It was the reference to that uniquely rapt attention which caught my eye when *The Mail & Guardian* was delivered that day. I paged through it as usual, scanning it for features demanding closer attention. The opening paragraph struck a chord. I was riveted as I read further – it explained so much. I stared out of the window for a long time when I'd finished reading. This wasn't something I should lock away in my drawer.

Claire should read it too.

I folded the paper neatly inside my briefcase and took it home to show her.

✳

MIND-BLIND

THE ENIGMA OF AUTISM

As soon as you enter a classroom at the Key School in Johannesburg, you know these children are different.

They don't look different. Just kids in shorts and T-shirts, busy with puzzles at their desks. But no one notices your arrival. No giggling or whispering to the boy next door. They finger the puzzle pieces with rapt attention. Their focus seems odd. They're more interested in the shape of the edges than in the picture they're trying to build. No hands up. No requests for help.

Self contained. Inward looking.

Mind-blind . . .

It struck a chord immediately. Amy was different. Claire and I had no basis for comparison because we didn't know any other children but we knew from that first afternoon that her behaviour wasn't normal. By coincidence, our first attempt at diversion after the inauspicious Anna-encounter involved a jigsaw. We'd bought a large colourful one that morning – jigsaws had played a prominent role in my solitary childhood. My mother had a jigsaw table in the lounge – we had an ongoing jigsaw project that lasted almost a decade. The one we bought for Amy was probably too complicated for a child her age but we weren't yet geared up to child development. We just hoped to keep her occupied until her mother arrived to rescue us.

I spilled the pieces on the carpet. Bright, disconnected chunks of painted cardboard. I propped the box against the table so she could see the picture she was trying to build. It was a farmyard scene. Cows and ducks and sheep. A blue pond. A cheerful farmhouse. I found the four corner pieces and put them in place on the table.

'Let's start with the pond. Find all the blue pieces and we can join them up,' I suggested.

'Find all the blue pieces,' echoed Amy. 'Join them up.' Amy could repeat everything you said to her. We soon learned that this was more a sign of dysfunction than a special skill. The words didn't mean anything to her. She didn't use them to guide her selection. It was disconcerting. She didn't look at the picture on the box. She didn't pick out the blue pieces of cardboard. She picked up random pieces and traced their shape with her finger. She managed to slot a surprising number in together – but it seemed irrelevant where they fitted in the bigger picture. She approached each fragment in isolation rather than as a part of a coherent whole.

I was fascinated – despite my resentment over the disruption to my weekend plans. I grew more and more absorbed with Amy's strange behaviour as our babysitting duties evolved into a regular feature. Claire and I had accumulated a significant number of questions about Amy by the time I came across the article. Predictably, Claire had made a list. We added to it every evening when Amy went home with Kate or Michael. We noted frequencies.

Repetitions. Patterns. But we didn't discuss our list with her parents – Claire and Kate had too complicated a relationship. Both of them are hypersensitive. Aware of their radical differences. Claire said they'd think we were passing judgement on their child. Criticising the way they brought her up. That's why I was pleased to come across the article – I was curious to see what it could tell me about Amy.

I didn't anticipate how much it would tell me about Claire.

The Key School is one of six South African schools which specialise in the education of children with autism – a lifelong, complex and devastating disability. Estimates of prevalence vary greatly. Recent small scale, but intensive studies, indicate higher numbers than earlier ones, as the criteria for autistic disorders has been widened considerably over the years. Estimates across the whole spectrum range from around 40 to 90 per 10 000 births – which means that it is not as rare as was originally thought. To put it in perspective – autism occurs more frequently than childhood cancer, is 4 times as common as cerebral palsy and 17 times more prevalent than Down's Syndrome.

Children with autism are different from those affected by other serious developmental disorders because they don't look handicapped. In her landmark book, Autism – Explaining the Enigma, Uta Frith comments. 'More often than not, the young autistic child strikes the observer with a haunting and somehow other-worldly beauty. It's hard to imagine that behind the doll-like image, lies a subtle and devastating defect, a defect as cruel on the child as it is on the family.'

I thought of Amy, with her delicate profile. Her pale face. Her fragility. Limbs like twigs. She looks dreamy sometimes – as if she's shrouded in mist. A wraith. She makes me think of *Swan Lake* – though she isn't graceful. She often knocks things over.

And I started to think of Claire . . .

The majority of people with autism are profoundly alone – cut off from normal social relationships. Although they can see the world around them, they're blind to what it means. They don't understand the nuances of language. Even if they're able to talk, they echo what they hear, rather than respond to what is said.

Autism was first recognised by Leo Kanner in 1943. The term is derived from the Greek word autos, which relates to self. The autistic person withdraws from social life into self and is unable to sustain normal relationships. Kanner noted three core characteristics.

- *Autistic aloneness – the inability to relate to people and situations. Anything that comes to the child from outside is shut out. They are self absorbed, with severe social, communication and behavioural problems. This is not the same as shyness – it's a mental rather than a physical aloneness.*
- *Obsessive insistence on sameness – the autistic person adheres to rigid, repetitive routines which lack apparent purpose. They tend to focus on a narrow topic of interest to the exclusion of everything else.*
- *Islets of ability – autistic children are sometimes in possession of splinter skills which stand out in marked contrast to their general level of achievement. A small percentage may have an outstanding vocabulary or phenomenal rote memory skills. Some are exceptionally musical, with perfect pitch and uncanny musical recall. Although characteristically clumsy, they can possess refined motor skills.*

A cascade of images. Snapshots. Falling like a pack of cards onto the table. I felt as if I'd suddenly mastered a foreign language. It was a revelation.

I recalled a recent weekend with Amy. She was holding a sheath of coloured paper. We wanted to encourage her to draw – I was spellbound by her drawing. But Amy never responded to a suggestion – it was as if she had her own agenda. She did the same thing every time we handed her the week's supply of paper. She shifted the papers, trying to get them in a perfect alignment. It was almost a ritual. It took ages because she was so clumsy. She kept dropping pages. Picking them up. Starting over. It drove me mad. I had to force myself not to do it for her. When they were perfect, she picked up the scissors. Held them awkwardly. Started to cut. This was what was remarkable. She cut the paper into strips. Thin strips, remarkable for their uniformity. She cut up the whole pile. Each strip looked equal – as if she'd measured them with a ruler. Her precision was mind-boggling. I couldn't have matched it.

But she lost interest as soon as she cut the final strip. It was a ritual aimed at nothing. She didn't seem to get any satisfaction out of doing it. She never looked at the strips. Didn't touch them.

Until she did it again next week . . .

It reminded me of Claire in the kitchen. Nowhere is her contrast to her sister more marked. Kate now asks us to stay for supper when we drop Amy. She always plays music while she cooks. She chucks in ingredients at random. Herbs and spices. Half a bottle of wine. The kitchen's in chaos by the time we eat – and the food is consistently terrible. Kate's whole house is a shambles. I'm not surprised Amy behaves

122

better when she's with us. Everything is always the same with us. We have a set routine for everything. Amy knows exactly what's going to happen next. Life with her mother must feel like a daily eruption of the local volcano.

Our town house has an open plan kitchen so I often watch Claire preparing meals while I'm working at the dining room table. She takes her recipe book out of the kitchen drawer. Puts it in place on the work surface. The same place every time – I'm sure it could be measured with a slide rule. She lines up all her utensils in a row in the order that she's going to use them. Claire owns a top of the range food processor but I've never seen her use it. She chops everything by hand. Perfectly symmetrical. Arranged in colours. Cubes of potatoes. Diced onion. Slivers of carrot.

Amy does the same with her crayons, now that I think about it. Before I read the article, it didn't strike me how much Claire and Amy have in common. Everyone can see they look alike – but even though I live with Claire, I didn't register the other similarities. On reflection, it's because their mutual oddness is on such a different scale. Claire seems merely eccentric. Her compulsive behaviour is mild enough to be dismissed as an idiosyncrasy. Only a ripple on the Richter scale. Amy's like a major fault line. A human San Antonio. She could reduce the western seaboard of North America to rubble when she gets into her swing.

But despite this disparity, there's a common thread – as if they're at different ends of a common spectrum. Subsequent paragraphs in the article supported this brand new thesis – it's amazing how a few thousand words can alter your perspective.

The Autistic Spectrum Disorder (ASD) is the most researched and validated syndrome of all developmental disorders. There are no physiological tests to determine whether a person has autism and a diagnosis is based solely on the observation of a number of characteristic behaviours. ASD can range from a person who is severely handicapped, exhibiting severely autistic behaviour through the area of mild and moderate autistic traits, then on to those affected by Asperger Syndrome who display very good intellectual ability but have certain prevalent autistic traits. Children in the latter group usually display only minimal learning disabilities and can often be absorbed into mainstream education. If teachers and parents are unaware of the characteristics of the syndrome, the condition can remain undiagnosed.

Could Claire be a milder variant of Amy? Could Claire's characteristic strangeness have a medical explanation? Claire's mother was dogmatically blind to the suggestion of any defects in her genetic pool. She would never have considered taking Claire to a doctor. Or a psychiatrist. She remained adamant that there was nothing wrong with Amy, despite the mounting evidence to the contrary. Claire isn't handicapped on the same scale – but that doesn't rule out autism. In fact, all people with Asperger's possess an average or above average intelligence – it's one of the criteria. The same is true for communication. An individual with Asperger's cannot display a clinically significant delay in language.

I'd never heard of Asperger's before that day and I know that was true for everyone we mixed with. It was as if I'd been handed a key to unlock a box of family secrets. I thought of Pandora. I was anxious about what I might learn as I poured over the insert on Asperger's Syndrome.

In 1944, Hans Asperger, an Austrian physician, published an account describing children with impaired social interactions and communication – intelligent, highly verbal, near-normal autistic children. Most autistic people achieve lower scores in verbal as opposed to non verbal skills tests but the reverse may be true of people with Asperger's. In 1989, Dr Christopher Gillberg formulated the following criteria for possible diagnosis.

I was riveted as I browsed through the list. Inability to interact with peers, coupled with a lack of desire to interact with peers. That had always been one of the differences I'd been aware of between Claire and me. I would have liked to join my colleagues for a drink. Claire didn't seem to notice that the office pub existed. All-absorbing narrow skills. I thought of her computer, her obsession with statistics. The ability to remember facts and figures that made her such an asset to Irving Life. Her inflexible routines. The lack of inflection in her speech. Her unexpressive face. Her lack of imagination.

Dr Gillberg could have used Claire as a case study.

It took me back to another urinal conversation I'd overheard. The urinal is an invaluable source of office information. People tend to overlook me. They carry on talking as if I'm invisible. I've noticed panic in their faces when they register my presence, as they scramble back through their conversation for comments that might have offended me. My position in the company unnerves them. I can see they're worried about what they might have said about my wife.

But everything they said about Claire that day was true.

'Christ,' complained Anderton. 'I'm exhausted. I've been closeted with Claire for over an hour. We're working on the Barlow's package. I get more reaction from the fucking computer than I do from her. She doesn't listen to what I'm saying. She doesn't register that I'm pissed off. And her voice. It drives me insane. It's so monotonous – I sink into a coma after about five minutes. There's no point in trying to make a contribution. It's all a one-way stream with her. I've tried making a few jokes. She doesn't react to sarcasm. I don't think she'd register if I had an epileptic fit. Or if I farted. She's impossible. I don't even notice that she's good looking any more.'

'I know what you mean,' said Ogalvie. 'She may be a mathematical guru but she's blinkered. She only considers textbook solutions. She threw my proposals out of the window – I don't think she heard a word I said in their defence.'

Anderton and Ogalvie are jealous of Claire – they want her job – but I must concede that there's an element of truth in what they said. Despite Claire's skills, her potential for promotion is limited. She won't go any higher at Irving's. I saw that as early as the AIDS project. Her work is meticulous. And accurate. Her weakness lies in predicting change. And AIDS is changing the demographics of the country. Turning them upside down. Claire's good at applying the lessons of the past. Not so good at predicting future trends – and that's an integral part of actuarial science. Even I have more imagination than she does. I'm always imagining what they might be saying about the things I say or do.

Claire seems impervious to office opinion.

But she wasn't impervious to *The Mail & Guardian* that evening. She read the article with the same intensity as I had. I'm not sure how I'd describe her reaction. I thought she might dismiss it as nonsense. Or be angry with me for suggesting that it might be relevant. She didn't discuss it with me that night but I had the feeling that she wasn't upset by what she'd read.

She seemed almost relieved.

Claire : Ice-blue. Triangular.

I couldn't get to sleep the night I read the article on autism. I have almost photographic recall of pages I've read recently so I could visualise the paragraphs, even after I switched off my bedside light. I reread them in my mind. Over and over.

I felt vindicated by what they had to tell me.

My mother said the same about a friend whose husband had been diagnosed with cancer. She said the diagnosis came as a relief. He'd been tired for so long. Frequently off work. Headaches. Lacklustre. No enthusiasm for anything. His colleagues thought he was neurotic so the diagnosis gave him credibility. People had to take his symptoms seriously once the doctor handed him a death sentence.

I knew I wasn't dying but somehow I felt empowered to learn that there could be a medical explanation for the things that made me so different from everyone else. Maybe it made me more interesting to myself. Less peculiar. As I lay in the dark bedroom, silent but for Tony's breathing, I felt comforted to think that there were other people as alien as me. It was like being granted membership to a secret society. There wasn't a long queue of people jostling for entry but I was glad to hear that it existed.

It made me feel less inadequate. It wasn't my fault. And it wasn't Amy's fault either.

I tossed and turned till morning filtered through the curtains. What was I going to say to Kate?

'Won't you tell her?' I asked Tony as I poured our pre-work coffee.

'Me?' said Tony, disbelieving. 'I can't possibly tell her. I don't think Kate's heard a word I've said from the day I met her. I remember how she and Michael looked at each other the night we went to dinner after we got back from Japan. I've never raised a single topic she's found interesting. I'm not always sure she'll recognise me if I pass her in the street.'

What he said was true. I sometimes thought it also applied to me. Despite the blood link. Despite the sudden acceleration in our contact since we'd started looking after Amy on a regular basis. Kate and I never discussed our mutual child. I had no idea what she thought about Amy's strangeness. She had to be aware of it. She looked permanently exhausted. I once heard her ask my mother if all children behaved like Amy sometimes.

I'm not an empathetic person but I felt sorry for Kate that afternoon as her daughter gave a high-decibel performance of the Amy-variations we'd come to dread. Refusing to eat. Walking on tiptoe. Twirling her hair. Flapping her hands. Screaming. Wedging herself into a ball underneath my mother's antique dresser. Her behaviour seemed so pointless. It drove us mad. It drove us out of my mother's house at the earliest opportunity.

It was only after Kate left Amy with us that we learned to tolerate her. We got involved. Uncharacteristically involved. We were interested in Amy. In the way she wouldn't look at us directly. Her abstracted gaze. By the random talents she'd occasionally display. And we were bowled over when suddenly she'd smile. Or reach out to take a hand. Or clamber into a lap. She seemed content to stay with us. She didn't bark and wag her tail when Kate came to fetch her. She was as impervious as Anna.

I was used to standing backstage, while Kate soaked up the limelight.

I was flattered by Amy's lack of preference.

*

Don't hate the messenger – that's an old adage about receiving bad news. Kate obviously hadn't heard it. Or she didn't believe it. She said she didn't believe that Amy was autistic either.

I could see she hated me for making the suggestion.

I brought the subject up in a most uncharacteristic way. Impulsively. I seldom act on impulse. Tony and I felt we had an obligation to tell Kate and Michael about the article we'd read – it went on to discuss the importance of early intervention in autistic education. We thought Amy should get professional help at the earliest opportunity.

But it's not an easy thing to tell your sister. Or your mother. I'd spent all week on the Net – and the more I learned, the more reluctant I became to share the information. Autism's not like asthma. Amy won't grow out of it. She won't make friends. Share a joke. Fall in love. It's hard to contemplate her future. And it's a long future. People with autism have a normal lifespan. Amy won't fall off the planet as she gets older. Kate and Michael will have to face the fact that she'll outlive them. Then who'll look after her?

It's daunting. I know because I've been there. To some extent. Amy's more extreme than me. I was a more passive child – as far as I can remember. I also knew that I was coming to conclusions far too quickly. I'm not a doctor. I was assuming a diagnosis cast in stone, triggered by a random article in the weekly newspaper. But the more I researched the topic, the more appropriate my conclusion seemed.

Perhaps I wanted it to be true. If it could be true for Amy, it could be true for me. All the latest research stresses the genetic link. I wanted to adopt Asperger's Syndrome as a scapegoat for everything that dissatisfied me about myself. I'd never go to a doctor. I couldn't face a string of questions. Intimate answers.

The next best thing was for Amy to go to a doctor.

So that's what I suggested. Out of the blue. With no preamble. As my father was carving the Sunday chicken. The thought had been buzzing for days like a persistent insect in the boundaries of my head. Somehow, I let it out. Translated it into words for everyone to hear.

'I think Amy's autistic,' I said. Baldly. Clinically. I must have sounded like the ice queen – I know they call me that at work.

'I think you should take her to a doctor,' I continued, filling the silence that had chilled everything around the table.

'There's nothing wrong with Amy,' said my mother. Predictably. Instinctively. She would have set a good example to a she-wolf, protecting her cubs from danger. 'Why on earth would she be autistic? What do you mean by autistic anyway? It's probably another of these modern buzzwords. Half the women at my book club claim their grandchildren are hyperactive. Or have occupational therapy or attention deficit or some other dreadful problem. Your generation's got a fixation about applying labels. They're just children. All of them behave badly sometimes. But they'll all grow up to be normal adults. Just like the four of you.'

Those were badly chosen words to conclude my mother's attempt to restore harmony to the lunch table. Neither of her daughters – nor her sons-in law – fitted that description. We didn't all belong on the autistic spectrum but we did span a wide range of behaviour patterns. Kate and Michael on one end – larger than life, bursting with vitality and confidence and talent. And Tony and me, reclusive in our upmarket cave, safe and sheltered from a world where we were misfits.

Amy was our only common thread.

Kate was angry. She exploded. She told me I didn't know

what I was talking about. To keep my crackpot diagnoses to myself. She said she didn't have time to sit around and listen to nonsense. She picked Amy up and stormed out of the house. Doors slamming. Engine revving. Wheels skidding on the gravel driveway.

She told me later she'd gone cold with fear when I spoke. She knew there was something seriously wrong with Amy. But no one had said anything before. She guessed her friends discussed it – Amy's behaviour was too extreme to overlook. But as long as no one said anything, she could tell herself it wasn't true. She brushed Michael aside when he tried to raise the subject.

It was the longest conversation Kate and I had ever had.

※

Kate said she wanted to push my words under the carpet. Into the darkest, dustiest corner where they couldn't see the sunlight. Where they couldn't put down roots and grow into a suggestion they'd have to confront and deal with. But she wasn't Amy's only parent. Michael wasn't as quick to wield a broom as Kate. He insisted that they take Amy to a doctor. Just to clear the air. Just for reassurance. Just in case . . .

My mother couldn't wait to pick up the phone to tell me what he had to say.

'I know you don't like me to phone you at work,' she started, 'but I felt you'd like to hear what happened at Amy's appointment. You were totally wrong about her. Kate and Michael have just dropped her off with me. Gallager says she seems perfectly normal for her age. Kate said he asked her a whole lot of questions about Amy's development and she did everything on time. Virtually on time. He says maybe she's a bit hyperactive but I'm sure she'll settle down once she starts school. I think it's probably because Kate and Michael have such irregular hours. Poor Amy doesn't know whether she's supposed to be awake or asleep. I'm sure that's why she's difficult sometimes.'

'Did they ask him about autism?' I asked.

'Oh, I don't know if they mentioned it specifically,' said my mother. Airily. Evasively. 'But Gallager didn't suggest it. And he's the doctor, after all. He sees so many children. I'm sure he'd be the first to pick up a problem.'

I didn't share my mother's confidence in Gallager. He was our family doctor. He'd been running the practice for at least twenty years. I doubt whether he keeps up with new opinions. I'm not certain that he's mastered email. He probably regards autism as a rare occurrence.

He'd never suggested that there was anything wrong with me . . .

'How long were they there?' I asked.

'Oh, I don't know exactly,' said my mother. She was very vague about the details. I think she felt they belonged under the carpet, along with my suggestion. 'But Gallager's always very thorough. He gave Amy a full examination. Kate said they had to hold her down – but children are always frightened of stethoscopes. They feel so cold when they touch your chest. And the doctor looks like an alien from outer space with the tubes protruding from his ears. And then there's that little light he shines in your eyes. And your ears. Amy doesn't like lights. Of course she'd make a bit of a fuss. But Gallager would have noticed if there was a problem. He's not one of these new-fangled young graduates with all their jargon and lightning diagnoses. He put her on Ritalin. That's what Sheila's granddaughter's on and it quietened her down straight away. I know you were just trying to help but you've really upset Kate. There was no need to say that about Amy.'

It took my mother quite a while before she was able to introduce autism into her vocabulary. She was reluctant to use the word. As if it was a witch's spell. Or a jinx.

As if saying the word might make my suggestion come true.

✳

Michael was more receptive to the seed I'd planted. He sounded ill at ease when he phoned and asked if he could buy me a cappuccino at the coffee bar across the road from Irving Life.

'Jesus, Claire,' he started, as I sat down at the small table in the corner. 'I feel bloody awkward meeting you here behind Kate's back. It's like I'm about to commit adultery. With her sister. It doesn't help that you look as if you just stepped out of a Hollywood blockbuster. Sisters-in-law are supposed to be plump and matronly with glasses.'

I just looked at him. I was always ill at ease with Michael. He was too theatrical for me. Very good-looking. Very physical. But he was over-the-top. Almost camp sometimes, despite his masculinity. He automatically played to his audience.

But I'd never been in the audience before. I only got his attention because of Amy.

'It's hard to explain how I feel about Amy,' he started. 'How I've always felt. From the moment she arrived. Maybe it's a sense of possession. She's mine – in a way that Kate will never be. Kate and I have always functioned independently. She doesn't need me in the same way that Amy does. I don't feel responsible for Kate. But I am responsible for Amy.'

I still didn't say anything. I'd be excommunicated as a priest. Banned forever as a Lifeline counsellor. I had no idea what to say. People didn't make a habit of telling me how they were feeling. But Michael wasn't daunted. He seemed determined to continue. I could see that he'd given a lot of thought to what he wanted to say.

'I love Amy. I can't tell you how much. I can't put it into words without sounding like Mills and Boon. But I love her. You'll have to take my word for it. And I'm worried about her. Because she's changed. It's like a regression. She was such a happy baby. She smiled and pointed. She knew my face. Responded to the games we played. But it's as if a curtain has fallen down between us. She under-reacts. Or over-reacts. Kate's not as aware of it as I am because she doesn't spend as much time with her as I do. Her career is bigger than mine so it's been logical for me to take the major role with Amy.'

'But Gallager said there wasn't a problem,' I ventured. Cautiously. I have zero experience in either medicine or childcare. I didn't want to be too dogmatic about my diagnosis.

'She actually behaved like a wild thing,' said Michael ruefully. 'I can see why he suggested she was hyperactive. But he only saw one side of her. Sometimes she's spaced out. Far away. I can't reach her. She won't even look in my direction. She seems totally unaware of what's going on around her. And she's speaking less and less. Instead of more and more. She's not reaching the same milestones as other children. But she looks blank rather than retarded. Perhaps I'm deceiving myself but I sometimes wonder if she's not a rocket scientist. In the closet. She sat beside me in the sandpit yesterday, pouring sand into a funnel. She just kept pouring. Watched it swirl and disappear. As if she was conducting an experiment. It was uncanny. Unnatural. Like Tommy. Did you see *Tommy?* The Who's rock opera. We put it on in my final year at Tech. Maybe you missed it. You don't come over as a disciple of rock opera. It was at the State Theatre. Maybe you were tempted?'

And he smiled at me. Quizzically. Directly. I felt my heart give an unfamiliar lurch. I'd never been the focus of Michael's charm before. He was very attractive. A lean, intelligent face. Warm brown eyes. Smiling especially for me.

I was flattered – but only for a moment. I put my heart firmly back into its usual place. I knew where I belonged. In the shallow end of the pool. With Tony. Where my feet could touch the ground and the water was clear and tranquil. Where I could see exactly what was coming next. I knew I'd drown in the deep end where Michael liked to swim. I wasn't made for waves that sweep you up and hurl you down at random. But when he smiled at me that morning, I caught a glimpse of what it might be like to go wherever the current took me.

I'd never take the risk. I came back to the crowded coffee bar. Back to the only reason he'd come to see me.

Back to Amy.

'I did see *Tommy*, actually,' I told him. I didn't tell him why. Kate and Michael were a well established item at the time. I went because he was in it. I'd heard conflicting reports about the show. I hoped Kate's attractive boyfriend would be a dismal failure. And I did come away from the theatre that evening with a sense of failure. But it wasn't Michael who'd failed. He dominated the stage as Tommy – the deaf, dumb, blind kid.

He sure played a mean pin-ball.

I was the one who felt a failure. I hated *Tommy*. I hated the music. I hadn't a clue what the play was about. It was a high-tech, special effects display of jumbled images. It seemed sacrilegious. High priests strumming heavy rock in church. Pilgrims worshipping at the feet of a huge icon of Marilyn Monroe, her famous white dress swirling up to show her panties. And Tommy. Bemused. Stranded. Fascinated by the lights and buzzing balls of the pinball machine. His uncanny ability to achieve scores right off the board. A random splinter skill.

Like Amy's cats . . .

I have the review of the play pasted in my book – it's really a combination book for Kate and Michael. Kate dominates because she's more versatile than Michael. South African theatre doesn't have the funds to finance the star-spangled musicals that are Michael's forte. *Tommy* was a low budget student production.

A standing ovation on opening night reflects the fact that the Drama Tech pulled out all the stops for their production of The Who's rock opera, Tommy. Built around the considerable talents of Michael

Templeton, the show runs like clockwork, with high tech touches that enhance and amplify the impact of the play. Considering the restrictions of their budget, the students have pulled off a remarkable achievement. The choreography is impressive, the singers talented – and the band kicks major ass, gluing the production together.

The play casts a look at humanity and its pitfalls. We are all wrestling with our inner demons. We all want to be what we are least. It's a remarkable play with a powerful message about exploitation of those least able to protect themselves. Written by The Who back in '69, it still has relevance today. The 20th anniversary performance at Radio City Music Hall in New York featured many top artists of the 80s and the play won 5 Tony Awards on Broadway. It was a big ask for Michael Templeton and his team from Pretoria Tech to pull off a production on this scale – and they've done it with style. Don't miss Tommy at the State Theatre this week.

'Tommy makes me think of Amy,' mused Michael. 'I watched Ken Russell's film on video recently. Oliver Reed. Jack Nicholson. I wonder if the world looks as chaotic to Amy as it did to Tommy. The lines keep coming back to me.' I watched his long, lean fingers drumming out a rhythm on the table as he hummed the words.

Tommy doesn't know what day it is . . .
I often wonder what he's feeling.
Has he heard a word I've said?
What is happening in his head?
How can he be saved?

'That's what today is all about,' he continued. 'There's another line that haunts me. The priests sing it in the church

139

as the wounded gather to touch the feet of Marilyn Monroe. *She's got the power to heal you.* After Kate stormed out on Sunday, you said you'd been researching autism on the Net. I've got to find a way to reach Amy. To get her back. What have you found out about autistic education in South Africa? Is there any hope that Amy can be rehabilitated?'

*

I made an appointment to see Linda Fenton – she's the psychologist at Unica – the school for autistic children in Pretoria. It's bigger and better equipped than the school in Jo'burg. I drove out to see her, armed with a sheaf of lists about Amy. Her behaviour. Our questions.

I needn't have bothered. I spent the morning talking about myself.

Linda Fenton is a busy woman. I had to wait nearly three weeks for an appointment. The school is seriously understaffed and under-financed. 'Children with autism require specialised, long-term education,' she explained. 'It's expensive – a low pupil-teacher ratio is essential if we hope to make some progress. There are huge demands on the education budget in South Africa so government subsidies are woefully inadequate and decreasing.'

She asked me why I thought Amy might be autistic. I told her about the article I'd read. I mentioned that it stressed the genetic link. And I found myself telling her all about myself. I'd never talked to anyone so intimately before. Not to Tony. Certainly not to Kate. Not even to my mother. It was as if a dam had broken. The words spilled out. I was helpless to stop them. I told her everything. All my inadequacies. I told her about Kate. About Tony. I even told her about sex and diabetes.

I can't explain where the words suddenly came from. Maybe it was her face. She was a tall woman in her late forties with a string of degrees behind her name. Her face seemed etched with compassion. She wasn't like my mother. She didn't say that I was talking nonsense. And she didn't pass judgement. I felt curiously relieved when I finished talking.

Perhaps my thoughts had some validity after all.

She suggested I read *Thinking in Pictures* – a book by Temple Grandin, a high achieving autistic adult. She thought some of Grandin's comments might strike a chord with me. She also gave me a questionnaire to take home to Kate and Michael. It was a weighty document – twenty-seven typed pages of detailed questions. I could see Kate was daunted when I handed it over. She phoned me later the same evening. Asked if she could come round to see us. She burst into tears the minute I opened the door.

'I don't know the answers to all these questions,' she sobbed. 'I feel so fucking useless. I don't know what to say. I have to describe my relationship with Amy. And her relationship with Mom and Dad. Even with you. What's your relationship like with Amy? I don't have a fucking clue. I just pick her up and take her home. And all her developmental milestones. Toilet training. Dressing. Zips. Lacing shoes. Can she tie a bow? How does she hold her scissors? Does she mind having her hair washed? Does she work with her face too close to the paper? Can she give messages? How does she react to sounds? Did she babble? Does she initiate conversation?'

She threw the document despairingly on the floor.

'I'm an awful mother!' she sobbed. 'My poor little girl. This is all my fault. I haven't paid her enough attention. What sort of mother can't remember what her baby did? Or when she did it? No wonder Amy's sick . . .'

For the first time in my life, I put my arms around her. Held her while she sobbed. Comforted her. I said I'd help her with the questionnaire. The four of us would fill it in together. Gather all our viewpoints. We'd give the most comprehensive picture possible of our little girl.

It was a major milestone.

And it's all because of Amy. I can't stop reflecting how much influence she's had. It's ironic. She doesn't seem aware of us as individuals but she's somehow shifted all our perspectives. It reminds me of my old kaleidoscope – my favourite childhood toy. The key fragments are still in place. Tony and me. Kate and Michael. All our parents. And Amy. She's shifted to the central role and we've all rearranged ourselves around her. Tony and I had always been outsiders – she's the one who's drawn us in. Cast us in roles we haven't played before. I'd never confided in anyone. And no one had ever confided in me. Or asked for my help. I felt empowered. For the first time in my life, I felt that I might be able to make a human contribution.

I think Tony felt the same. Our relationship with Amy had shifted in a subtle way. And our relationship with each other. It seemed as if the kaleidoscope was still turning. We'd been interested in Amy – because of autism, I suppose. It's a fascinating syndrome with all its contradictions. We'd started off as observers. Noting down the facts. Recording trends. But it's become personal now, as we've got to know her. We've learned to recognise her moods. We try to choose the things she likes. Her smile's a reward we value highly. Any response is good – any indication that she remembers something from the day before.

Tony and I are very fond of Amy. Perhaps we even love her.

I know her parents love her. Their lives revolve around her. So do ours. But our focus is different. Even their own reactions to Amy are in sharp contrast. Michael's searching for salvation – he's determined to find a cure. To make her better. He hasn't yet accepted autism as a lifelong label. Michael's focus is on Amy's future. Kate's is on her past. Why it happened. She's worked her way back to the viral infection she had during her early pregnancy – I've found a lot about neonatal influences on the Net. She's obsessed with the things she did. Or didn't do. She's taken personal responsibility for a medical condition.

No one can persuade her that it's not her fault.

I found her curled up on a chair with a book one afternoon. Tears pouring down her face. 'What's wrong?' I asked, fear clutching at my heart. 'Has something happened to Amy?'

'I'm what's happened to Amy,' she sobbed. 'Look at this book.' She passed it to me, blindly. I looked at the cover. *The Empty Fortress*. Bruno Bettelheim. I'd heard of it – it was highly influential when it was first published.

'He says children are autistic because of their mothers,' Kate wept, despairingly. 'They don't give them enough love and attention. No support. They don't comfort them when they cry. I used to leave Amy crying in her cot while I soaked up the limelight. She must have felt abandoned. I didn't bond properly with her when she was a baby. The refrigerator mother – it's me he's describing. Me and my fucking career. I don't deserve to have a baby.'

'This book's been totally discredited,' I assured her. 'It's cruel nonsense. And no one could ever describe you in terms of a refrigerator – it's the direct opposite of everything you are. Neither you nor Michael is cold. It would be more relevant if I'd been Amy's mother. Amy has a genetic defect. Autism has nothing to do with bad parenting. All the latest research stresses that.'

But you can't tell Kate anything. She doesn't deal in factual medical opinion. Life for her is a turmoil of emotion. And her predominant emotion with regard to Amy is guilt. Guilt's a destructive emotion. The Oxford defines it as a mental obsession with the idea of having done wrong. It's damaged her relationship with Michael. Even Tony and I seem closer than they are now.

It wasn't always an obsession of its current proportions. It's got worse over the last two years. Ever since Amy's fourth birthday. I don't know what happened between them – Kate's confidences extend only to her daughter's education. I can't explain what's gone wrong with her marriage.

It must be linked to Amy. She's the catalyst for everything that happens in our family circle.

*

Kate and Michael asked me to go with them to Pretoria on the day that Amy was to be evaluated by the school's psychiatric team. 'Please come,' said Kate. 'We need you. I'm scared I'm going to give all the wrong answers. I'll get emotional and lose my temper. I need you to concentrate on what they're saying. You can make a list. I'll feel more secure if you're there. It will help us get a better deal for Amy.'

I could understand why they were nervous. This wasn't going to be a fifteen minute session with Gallager and his stethoscope. There's no physical test for autism. We'd already submitted the daunting questionnaire covering her developmental milestones. They'd caused sufficient concern to warrant an interview. Amy faced a lengthy period of observation by a team of specialists. A psychiatrist. The school principal. A senior teacher. A psychologist. An occupational therapist. A speech therapist. I could sense that Kate and Michael were terrified about what they might learn about their little girl.

We were silent as we drove out along the highway. I sat in the back with Amy. Neither of us is noted for small talk. And Kate and Michael said nothing. Not to her. Not to me. Not to each other.

The tension in the car was tangible.

It increased as we approached the school. Our appointment was at ten o'clock. It was break and the playground was full of children. Under watchful supervision. A playground at a school for children with autism is so quiet. It wasn't gloomy. Just quieter than you'd expect. We saw a boy on the swing. Backwards and forwards, higher and higher. All alone. Not calling out to anyone. Another boy was lying on top of the slide, completely still, curved in towards himself — there was a predominance of boys. Autism is much more common in boys. Other children were walking around. A girl twirling a plant. A boy going through the motions of a kung-fu fighter. Another jumping on a trampoline. None of them seemed unhappy but there was no interaction. No one was telling anyone else what he was up to. The entire playground seemed self-absorbed.

It was very disconcerting. Amy was the only one who didn't notice.

We sat down in front of the panel. Like three delinquent children. I left the questions to Kate and Michael. And the answers. I wrote everything down in my careful script. Meticulously. I left nothing out. I was well-schooled in precision after my years at Irving Life. We left Amy with them and walked around the school. Watched the teachers, busy in their classrooms. Got a feel for what the school could offer Amy.

Kate was silent as the teacher led us from one classroom to the next. Different age groups. Different levels of disability. Art. Music. Occupational therapy. It was a varied, comprehensive programme. We were left in a small lounge – she brought us a tray of tea to pass the time. Until the jury came back to give the judge their verdict. Kate looked like an unexploded bomb. Her hands shook as she took the cup of tea I poured her. It spilled into the saucer. Onto her dress. Perhaps the heat triggered a reaction.

Because she started to talk. Michael and I listened. Helplessly. We knew it would be impossible to make her change her mind.

'Amy's not coming to this school,' she said. 'Whatever they say. However fucking autistic they decide she is. Did you see some of those children? You can see they're seriously retarded. Mentally deficient. They can't do a thing for themselves. They can't talk at all. Not a single sentence. Not one coherent thought. It's impossible to educate a child

146

like that. I won't put Amy in a class with them on a daily basis. They'll drag her down. Make her like them. She'll be given a label that she'll have to carry around forever. She'll be categorised and people will give up on her.'

'I know all about labels,' she continued. 'They stuck one on me in my first year at high school. It said arty. Non-academic. The opposite of my sister. No one had any expectations that I might be good at anything other than drama. And I went along with it. I believed my label so I never tried to get into a different category. Everyone's response to me has always been governed by the label I was given. I won't have Amy labelled. And that's that.'

Kate's words struck a chord with me. I'd always been the clever one. The maths fundi. The ice-princess. And Tony – everyone wrote him off as boring. A monochrome. Even I hadn't questioned it. I never asked Tony for his opinion. I assumed he didn't have one. I could understand Kate's point of view – even though I'd found the school impressive.

We felt as if we'd run a marathon by the time we were called through for the final session. The principal shifted through the pile of notes on the desk in front of her. Sorted them into order. There was obviously a set procedure that she had to follow. Michael took Kate's hand and held it tightly as they listened to the facts about ASD. The Autistic Spectrum Disorder. What it was. The result of disordered brain development and function. And what it wasn't.

'Autism has nothing to do with bad parenting,' she told them. 'It's not a psychological or emotional disorder. Children with ASD don't choose to misbehave.' She went on to stress the broadness of the spectrum. 'It's impossible to generalise about people with autism,' she told us. 'The spectrum extends from university professors to severely handicapped people who will require institutionalised care for the rest of their lives.'

She introduced us to the common thread that links them all.

The triad of impairments . . .

Impairment in reciprocal social interaction. Doesn't approach people for help. Lack of awareness of feelings. Poor eye contact. Impairment in communication. Appears deaf. Failure to initiate and sustain conversation. Abnormal pitch. Restricted, repetitive patterns of behaviour. Impaired imagination. Distressed by change. Motor stereotypes. Hand flapping. Spinning. And so on. And so on . . .

We didn't look at each other. They were describing Amy.

'At what stage were you sure that there was something wrong?' she asked Kate gently.

Kate looked back at her. Took a deep breath. Seemed to take a decision. She reached into her handbag and pulled out a crumpled sheet of paper. She smoothed it out and placed it on the table in front of the principal. Michael looked staggered as he leaned forward to have a look. It was obviously the first time he'd seen it.

It was my cat, Anna. It was nearly a year since I'd given Kate the drawing. I'd seen how much it upset her so I'd never referred to it again. I'm not good at initiating conversation.

It's a weakness I share with Amy.

＊

Amy's drawing confirmed the conclusion that had already been reached by the panel who'd observed her in a variety of contexts. A unanimous conclusion. Amy's behaviour met the necessary criteria for a diagnosis of early infantile autism. Because of her low verbal score and language delay, she didn't fit the criteria for Asperger's Syndrome. She wasn't as lucky as I am.

Kate and Michael were devastated.

It was different for Tony and me. We continued to be fascinated by Amy – far more than if she'd been a normal little girl, trotting off to playschool with her peers. We wouldn't have had any interest in stick-men drawings of mummy and daddy and the dog next door. But we were riveted by Amy's growing cat collection.

Her ability was uncanny. She could capture stillness or movement with equal acuity. She never used a rigid outline. Broken agitated lines suggested Anna's speed. Her agility. The lines grew thick and heavy when she caught the cat asleep. Her drawings seemed to exhibit a basic awareness of the form and structure of a cat. They could only be the result of observation – she had no knowledge of anatomy.

Her sense of proportion captivated me. She had an incredible visual sensitivity for detail. In the same way my ear can distinguish the minutest variation in tone, she could produce sketches of Anna with almost photographic precision. The gap between her eyes. Oval, almond eyes, positioned roughly halfway between the top of her ears and chin. Petal-shaped ears. Her heartlike face – quite small in relation to the rest of her body – statistically, the head of a cat should fit into the length of the body about four times, excluding the tail. Straight front legs, tapering to delicate fore-paw – contrasting with the ham-bone angle of her hindquarters.

The drawings were remarkable. I spent hours on the Net – I wanted to find out how rare her talents were. Tony browsed through the bookshop shelves. He bought a copy of Darold Treffert's book. *Extraordinary People*. Amy certainly fitted the description.

'Maybe she slots somewhere into the Savant Syndrome,' suggested Tony. 'It says it's a condition where someone with a major intellectual handicap has a special island of brilliance. A paradox. Ability and disability – existing side by side.'

We read everything we could find about the topic. We learned that child musicians are not uncommon but a study, done as early as 1926, was unable to locate a single child under twelve whose drawings had artistic merit. Savants more frequently exhibit musical genius. We read about Blind Tom – a sixteen-year-old slave with a vocabulary of less than a hundred words. His musical repertoire was astounding. Over five thousand catalogued pieces. He gave a performance for the president in the White House in 1849 when he was only eleven years old.

Apparently his mother was bought by a colonel in Georgia – he had daughters who practised their sonatas on the piano within hearing of the boy. Late one night, the colonel heard music coming from his drawing room. He found the four-year-old blind boy playing a Mozart sonata. The boy could play a complicated piece of music, note for note, after listening to it only once. I could hardly believe it.

'A statistical study was carried out in London in 1986,' Tony told me, always interested in facts and figures. 'Five musical savants were tested and their scores compared with a control group of normal children who were proficient on the piano. They rated musical competence – timing, rhythm, complexity of invention, modulation. And the savants came out on top.'

It made me think of Dustin Hoffman's *Rainman* – he could remember random numbers. From the telephone directory. In the casino. There was no logical reason to explain it. He just could. The musical savant plays brilliantly without understanding how he does it. It's like being good at maths. Both music and maths have predictable structural patterns. The savant seems to have unconscious access to these skills.

I was fascinated. I'm not a savant but I do have skills beyond the norm in maths and music. And Treffert stresses that while the music of the savant is impressive in terms of structure and accuracy, it's devoid of expression and innuendo. Wooden.

That's what my music teacher used to say about my efforts.

Artistic skills like Amy's were far rarer. I read Lorna Selfe's book on Nadia, based on research carried out at the Child Research Unit at the University of Nottingham in 1973. Nadia was diagnosed with early infantile autism. Extremely limited language. Echolalia. By six, she could only use a few limited phrases, interspersed with unintelligible jargon. She seemed withdrawn and isolated.

Like Amy.

But Nadia could draw – she also had that in common with Amy. Her drawings were phenomenal, dating from an even earlier age than Amy's. Selfe and Newson, her co-worker, had analysed, categorised and rated twenty-four thousand 'pictures of mummy', drawn by children throughout England for a competition. Nadia's drawings stood out among them. The hypothesis that Selfe puts forward to explain this seems logical to me. It revolves around compensation. Savants in any field are characterised by unusual rote memory skills. The artistic savant has access to a complex picture lexicon. A huge memory bank of shapes and images. Proportions and dimensions. Selfe postulates that their superior visual skills are linked to their limited verbal ability. All of us use visual imagery as our initial language. As we learn to talk, we use language as a form of shorthand. It supplants our visual memory which gradually decays through lack of use.

Amy had fewer and fewer words at her disposal. Perhaps it was a trade-off. She became hypersensitive in a narrow, feline channel. It's not unusual for these people to specialise in certain subjects. I learned of international examples. Steven Wiltshire is a British phenomenon. He's severely autistic and his work concentrates almost exclusively on architecture. At ten, he drew what he referred to as a London alphabet. Drawings of buildings from Albert Hall to the London Zoo. His sense of proportion and perspective is astonishing.

I poured over a catalogue of Yamamura, Japan's famous insect artist. Nadia's preference was for horses, although her focus wasn't as exclusive as Amy's cats. I even found another feline addict. Gottfried Mein. He was known as the Cat's Raphael. His work dates back to 1768. A stumbling cretin, with large rough hands. Totally illiterate. One of his paintings sold for a thousand pounds sterling as recently as 1971.

Extraordinary People is a fascinating book but I didn't lend it to Kate. I wasn't sure how she'd react. Anything remotely connected to autism was a minefield in those early days.

✳

The Christmas present was Tony's idea.

He felt we could be withholding vital information from Kate and Michael if we kept the drawings to ourselves. Amy only drew her cats at our house. Maybe Anna was an essential stimulus. We had seven drawings. We'd filed them as meticulously as usual. According to date. Not to subject matter. They were all of Anna in a variety of domestic situations. The first showed her angry, with arched back and bristling fur. As she'd been the first day that Amy saw her. Her recall was remarkable. It seemed that she didn't need to return to the original – a single exposure was sufficient to print the image in her mind forever.

'It's wrong that Kate and Michael haven't seen these drawings,' Tony argued when I said we should leave them safely out of sight. 'I've studied her cats in the finest detail. I believe her talent goes beyond mere motor reproduction. I think she should be actively encouraged by someone who knows more about art than we do. So she can reach her full potential. It's wrong to leave her parents in the dark.'

Then he came up with his suggestion. 'Why don't we have them framed? It'll solve the problem of what to get Kate for Christmas.' We always spent Christmas day with my parents. Tony's mother came too. And Michael's. We started with a champagne breakfast, followed by a traditional ceremony around the tree. My mother spent hours decking the halls with boughs of holly. All the Christmas trimmings. Her collection of decorations dates back to our early childhood. Ornaments that Kate and I had made at school. Kate's contribution far exceeded mine – I've never been creative. We put all our presents under the tree and my father donned a Santa hat and handed them out. We watched and applauded as each gift was unveiled.

Tony was pleased with his idea. He seldom made a contribution to family occasions. Even when he got to know them better. He was a quiet man, regardless of the setting. We're both quiet when Kate and Michael are around – they're major competition when it comes to making conversation.

We took Amy's drawings to a framer at Hyde Park. He'd recently framed a beautiful photograph of Amy for my mother. Captured her wistful charm. We'd all had copies made – they featured prominently in each family lounge. He gave us advice with regard to positioning each drawing to maximum effect. He arranged them in chronological order. He looked very sceptical when he heard Amy's age. Tony sounded like a proud father, bragging to the teachers. He spent a fortune on the frame but it was worth it. We were both delighted when we collected the final product. We wrapped it with our usual care. We were very pleased with ourselves when we managed to buy wrapping paper featuring cats in Christmas gear. We felt an unfamiliar thrill of anticipation as we set out to join the gathering of the clan on Christmas morning.

We usually gave everyone a gift pack from Woolworths.

We were the first to arrive. Kate and Michael were always late – it must be a genetic defect, inherited from his mother.

We piled our presents under the tree beside my mother's.

'That looks exciting, darling,' she said, as I placed the large rectangle carefully at the back of the pile. Tony and I exchanged glances. We could hardly wait to see their faces when Kate took off the wrapping. We were impatient for the others to arrive so my mother could get the proceedings underway. It would be ages before we reached the finale.

Christmas is the highlight of my mother's year. I've never spent a Christmas away from home. It's always been a major occasion in the family calendar. Everything happens in exactly the same way each year – but it's a tradition I wouldn't like to change. It always starts with paper hats and kisses at the door. Then Dad opens the champagne and Mom brings in the hot mince pies. They're delicious – light pastry, rich in butter, high in calories. And after that, there's a Christmas singalong. It's a tradition inherited from my grandmother – all of us are musical. We take our seats around the piano – it's the only time I ever play for other people. My mother persuaded me to do it for Granny when I was a little girl and it's continued ever since. My repertoire moves from Christmas carols to Boney-M. Tony's the only one who doesn't sing along with gusto. He's too shy to sing in public. His mother was also reticent at first but now adds her thin soprano to the chorus.

Even Amy sang that year. Kate and Michael urged her on. She was dressed in red gingham and looked so pretty. Some of the family enthusiasm seemed to rub off on her – she had more colour in her cheeks than usual. Her face lit up as she clapped her hands and stomped her feet, just like her parents. The three of them got up and danced when I got to Jingle Bells. Everyone called for an encore and we went through the chorus three times in succession.

We were flushed with pleasure as we settled down around the tree with Father Christmas. We all smiled at Amy as she pulled the paper off her presents. It was a lovely day – until Dad got to our present. 'The big one's for you Katie,' he said as he handed it over. It was heavy. We were afraid she'd drop it. We watched her face as she cut the ribbon and pulled the paper off.

Amy's cats, unveiled at last . . .

There was a chorus of exclamations when we said she was the artist. No one could believe it. They all crowded round to get a closer look. All talking at once.

'It was Tony's idea,' I told them. 'He chose the frame and placed the drawings. They're all in chronological order. I just had them lying around in a file at home. He thought of framing them.' I was more talkative than usual. Success had gone to my head.

I slowly realised that Kate was less talkative than usual. In fact, she was absolutely silent. She was the only one who hadn't raved about the drawings. Apart from Amy. Kate's face was as blank as her daughter's as she stared at her handiwork. Even my mother noticed.

'Are you all right darling?' she asked her. 'Aren't the drawings wonderful? Isn't it amazing to think that Amy did them all by herself?'

But Kate remained silent as she looked at our work of art. And then she burst into tears . . .

'I hate this!' she sobbed. 'These fucking cats! It's been such a lovely day and now it's spoiled! Claire's trying to turn Amy into a freak show. I just want her to go to play-school with the others. I want to stick funny pictures on my fridge with magnets. This looks as if I stole it from the National Gallery. I won't have it on my wall. I wish Amy could be like everyone else's children. I don't want a fucking genius. It's all because of Claire! I wish you'd kept your bloody genes to yourself!'

She picked up the frame and threw it down with all the force that she could muster. Stormed out and slammed the door. The picture fell heavily onto the tiled floor. The glass smashed. Splintered into what seemed a thousand fragments.

An appalled silence settled on the room.

✳

I'm not an emotional person. Kate's the family specialist in highs and lows. I don't remember feeling angry with her before. I'd resented her – resented all the skills she showed that I was lacking – but resentment's a quieter emotion than anger. It burns on a lower heat. Perhaps it burns for longer but the intensity's not that great. I switched my emotions up a gear when Kate smashed Tony's picture. All my plates were operating on high that Christmas morning. My simmering resentments boiled over into rage. I felt it coursing through my bloodstream, heating even my most distant corners.

If I'd had a gun, I would have shot her through the heart.

I felt sick with disappointment as we swept up the broken glass. Tony didn't say a word but his hands were shaking as he held out the dust tray to receive the remnants of our present. His brain child. His special tribute to Amy.

The whole family was shattered by Kate's performance.

Michael brought her round on Christmas evening to apologise for what she'd done. She looked awful. Face scrubbed raw from crying. Michael pushed her over the doorstep.

'Kate would like to apologise to you both for what happened this morning,' he started.

She burst into tears.

'I'm sorry!' she wept. 'I'm so, so sorry. I wish I could make you understand how sorry I am. I wanted to die when I got to the car and thought coherently about what I'd done. What I'd said. I wanted to come back but I couldn't face you. After everything you've done. For Amy. For Michael. And especially for me. I've taken advantage of your help and now I've thrown it in your faces. It's such a special present. I know how much time you must have spent getting everything together. I'm sorry. Please forgive me. I'm so sorry.'

Tony said nothing. He shifted awkwardly from foot to foot. I couldn't think of anything to contribute. Michael came to our rescue.

'We're all upset,' he said. 'Claire, why don't you make us each a cup of coffee? And I'll go and get some glasses. Raid Tony's wine rack. I think we could all do with a couple of glasses of that *Thelema* you gave us last time we came to dinner. Kate, why don't you and Tony take a seat and talk this through?'

I watched them sit down opposite each other as I switched on the kettle. And I saw Michael listening as he pretended to dust the spotless glasses on the shelf beside the wine rack.

Kate started uncharacteristically slowly. 'I want to try to

explain my reaction,' she told him. 'It's important that you understand that it wasn't a personal attack on you. However it sounded. I never think before I talk. I did the same the day Claire first suggested Amy might be autistic. I panic when I hear something I don't want to hear. Something that might be true. I know Amy's drawings are amazing but I can't bear to look at them. To me, they don't represent a real talent. They emphasise the extent of her dysfunction. I keep praying this will go away. Just disappear. That I'll wake up and find she's not autistic after all. Those cats underline everything that's wrong with Amy.'

Tony looked at her and cleared his throat. I knew how strongly he felt about the drawings. For once, he decided to say what he was thinking.

'I can understand that you might feel like that,' he answered. 'And it doesn't matter about the picture. It's only the glass that's broken. I can fix it if you change your mind. But I want to explain why I did it. You haven't looked at the drawings closely. At the details. The incredible accuracy of her recall. It was my idea to have them framed. It's not fair to blame Claire. She wanted to keep them in the file. It was me who thought that you should see them.'

'I don't blame either of you,' said Kate, on the brink of tears again. 'I'm the one who's in the wrong. But I'm so scared. I don't want Amy to hit the headlines because of the drawings. I know they're exceptional – but they're also abnormal. It takes me back to *Venus*. I had a small part in that in my first year at Wits. I don't know if you've heard of Saartjie Baartman. The Hottentot Venus. A young black woman from the Cape who was taken to Europe by a British navy doctor at the beginning of the century. Her remains have just been returned to South Africa in recognition of the wrong that was done. How she'd been exploited. No one saw her as a person. She was seen only as a freak. Because of her pendulous breasts. Her huge backside. Her blackness. She became a celebrity only because she was abnormal. I couldn't bear the same thing to happen to Amy. What if someone sees these drawings? Tells a journalist? I know what the media can do – it's part and parcel of my career. I don't want Amy in the limelight because of a freakish talent. It can't be called talent when she doesn't know she's using it.'

Tony didn't cave in and agree. I hadn't realised the strength of his feelings before that night. He shook his head. 'I think you're wrong,' he said. 'I've heard other people say that the public recognition of autistic talent is exploitation – that they're not really creative, with regard to either art or music. They echo rather than create. They're just mimicking something that they've heard or seen before. But even if that's true, it doesn't make their skills any less remarkable. You and Michael both have talent so perhaps you see things from a different perspective to me. You have no idea what it's like to always take the back seat. I've never been in the limelight. Despite my job. Only my mother thinks I'm wonderful. I don't think it's right to pretend that Amy doesn't have this talent – or skill, if you prefer it. It's part of what makes her who she is.'

Michael and I had got no further with the wine and coffee. We were open eavesdroppers. It was strange to hear Tony speak his mind. And equally strange for Kate to pause and think before she answered.

'I'm sorrier than ever,' she said slowly. 'I've underestimated you. I don't think I've ever really listened to you before tonight. I've done exactly what you said. Kept you in the background. Because you're quiet. Because you wear a suit. Even because you're an actuary. God knows what an actuary is – I've never made the slightest effort to find out. But I've been wrong. I don't agree with what you say about Amy but that doesn't mean I'm right. Perhaps I'll change my mind. You've made me think. I know how much time you spend on Amy. And so does Claire. I owe so much to both of you. I'm so sorry I've never said it before.'

Then she reverted to Kate-like behaviour. She got out of her chair and walked over to Tony. Threw her arms around his neck. Held him tightly. Burst into tears. I watched as his arms moved up awkwardly to pat her back.

Tony's face isn't expressive but I suspect his heart lurched when she did that. Like mine, the day Michael came to discuss Amy with me for the first time. Nothing will come of either occasion. Kate and Michael are in a different league from us. But I wonder if Tony and I have the same dream. As we lie in our separate beds. Side by side. Perhaps Kate sometimes crosses Tony's mind. Like Michael flits through mine. Mild delinquent thoughts.

We both know we're already in the place that's best for us.

Michael wasn't uppermost in my thoughts on the evening that followed the Christmas gift fiasco. I was haunted by Kate's genetic accusations. She'd apologised for them. Again and again. We both knew the blame she'd cast was nonsense. But I still felt guilty. I'd always resented Kate. Wished she could have some insight into what it was like to be me. The lesser sister. And it seemed that the gods had been listening after all. They'd given her Amy.

And Amy's so much more myself than I am.

I handed in my resignation at Irving Life. I was determined to launch a rescue bid for Amy.

A glimpse of the future?

Tony : Sepia. Background blended.

Thou shalt not covet thy neighbour's wife . . .

I'm not overly familiar with the Bible but I have a schoolboy recollection of the Ten Commandments. There's no specific reference to your wife's sister – and even if there were, no impartial jury would find me guilty.

I don't covet Kate. I don't wish I'd married her instead of Claire. I'd hate to live with someone so unpredictable. It would be tantamount to building a house in the path of a tropical hurricane. I don't have the stamina. Even a family lunch date is exhausting. But that doesn't preclude me from knowing she's gorgeous. Not classically gorgeous. Not like Claire. I've led a closeted life and I can state, without the shadow of a doubt, that Kate's the most glamorous, exciting person to ever cross my path.

I hoped she'd be bowled over by my present. I suppose it crossed my mind that she might kiss me. It wasn't an outrageous expectation – she seemed to kiss everyone else. But she never noticed me. The present was an attempt to register my presence. There was no element of physical desire in my fantasies of Kate – I'd look away and flinch if she took her clothes off. It was recognition that I wanted. Despite the hours I'd spent on her daughter, Kate had never given any indication that she knew I existed.

It was a big moment for me when it happened – when she put her arms around my neck and kissed me. It wasn't just a formal peck. She didn't pull away. It threw me totally off balance – because it happened nearly nine hours later than I'd anticipated. The circumstances were entirely different from the ones I'd imagined when I planned my strategy.

I was devastated by her initial reaction. I'd expected gratitude. I thought she'd be delighted. Even overwhelmed. Amazed at what her mystery child had been up to on the quiet. Her anger was totally unexpected. My predominant emotion was embarrassment. How could I have misread the situation so badly? I didn't know where to look. I've never been at ease with Claire's family – I couldn't look them in the eye. I knew they'd all be feeling sorry for me. I'd been hoping for praise. Not pity. I couldn't wait to get away.

Getting Kate's attention wasn't my only motive for framing Amy's drawings. I'm seldom really committed to a cause but I feel very strongly about this issue. Amy has a talent far beyond the norm and I believe it deserves recognition. By the people who care about her. Public accolades won't mean anything to Amy but I think we can be proud of her in private.

I know Kate understood. And I could see her point of view. I hadn't thought of the media. They'd love Amy. Not only because of her talent. They'd also snap her up because her mother has a high profile in the world of theatre. And because Amy's beautiful. Those three factors would be a winning combination for the media – but they'd be a brand new triad of impairments for Amy. It was strange that I'd found the words to plead my cause. I'm not accustomed to taking the role of orator. I felt I'd made my case – like an attorney on LA Law.

But the strangest aspect of that evening wasn't the fact that I was talking. I admit it was unusual, considering the topic – my eloquence is normally confined to banking issues. It was the direction of my words that surprised me. I realised I wasn't saying them for Kate. I didn't really care what she thought of me. I was explaining myself to Claire.

I was touched by the way she sprang to my defence that morning. Claire seldom reacts to anything – on the surface anyway. I know there's a huge chasm between public sentiment and private feelings but Claire's as cool as ice, no matter what the crisis. She lost her cool that morning when Kate threw down our gift and stormed out into the driveway. It's the first time in all our years of marriage I've seen her lose her temper.

'How dare she do this?' she almost shouted as she bent to help me sweep up the shards of shattered glass. 'How dare she? She hasn't even bothered to take a look at the drawings. You went to so much trouble. She hasn't thanked you. She hasn't even praised Amy. How dare she do this?'

Her voice was taut with anger.

Her reaction probably came as more of a shock to her parents than Kate's tantrum. Kate's tantrums were standard procedure – par for the course – but Claire's vehemence was a surprise, especially to me. She was furious. On my behalf. It lessened Kate's rejection of my carefully chosen present. It made me want to tell her why I felt so strongly about Amy's talent. I think she'd guessed. Discarded the initial opposition she voiced when I put forward my proposal. We hadn't discussed it any further. Debate wasn't a feature of my life with Claire.

But I wanted to explain myself. To justify the stand I'd taken in the light of Kate's unexpected opposition. I woke up early the next morning, the day after Christmas. I looked across at Claire as she lay sleeping. I could hear her quiet breathing. Her slim outline was covered only by a sheet. It was already hot. Temperatures rise quickly in December. As they'd risen as we sat in our family circle around the tree the day before.

It was strange to think I'd been the catalyst for all that had been said and done since then.

My feelings for Claire have slowly gained an extra dimension. I knew I was lying beside the most important person in my family circle. In my life. My mother's out of the competition. I could sense that everyone at the office thought I was lucky – based purely on Claire's appearance. And on my social limitations. But Claire's beauty was irrelevant to me. I was simply pleased that she'd taken my side. That she was upset by Kate's reaction.

Amy had upgraded my role as Claire's husband. It didn't seem a sinecure any longer. I felt I had more relevance than usual – to all Claire's family.

No one would ever forget my Christmas contribution.

✳

Apart from the central players, no one has any idea of the truth about a marriage. Claire's sudden resignation prompted a round of speculation at Irving Life. So you're a bit of a stallion on the side, Tony. Nudge, nudge. Wink, wink. They all thought she was pregnant. We didn't disillusion them. Neither of us has a confidant at the office. We'd never mentioned the demands of our existing child. No one knew about our involvement with Amy.

I was as surprised as the rest of the staff when Claire told me her decision – surprised enough to ask her why.

'Amy's not making any progress. I don't think any of her teachers really have any idea how to help her.' That's all she said. I didn't press the point because I agreed. Kate remained predictably determined to avoid a school specifically geared to children with disabilities. She became a devotee of various home-school bibles. Claire persuaded her to consign Bruno Bettelheim and his bonding theory to the dustbin. But the new discipleship was just as bad. She seemed attracted to any theory that saw mothers as the enemy.

Holding Therapy – the mother has to forcibly hold the child – in order to reverse the lack of bonding that made the child autistic in the first place. Kate's very tactile. We could see that it broke her into pieces when Amy wouldn't hug her, when she flinched and pulled away. But her efforts at holding therapy were a dismal failure. Amy went berserk. Kicked and screamed and lashed out in all directions. It destroyed Kate.

Michael made her throw Holding Therapy into the bin along with Bruno.

Claire downloaded an article on behaviour modification. Pioneered in Los Angeles by Ivor Lovaas, the treatment changed the focus of therapy from cause to conduct. It made much more sense to a results-oriented person like Claire. Instead of trying to understand the reasons for autistic behaviour, the Lovaas technique aims to reinforce positive behaviour patterns, through one-on-one inter-reaction between therapist and child. Lovaas reported progress with some children by creating a highly structured environment, using the repetition and consistency that's an integral part of the autistic personality. Some autistic parents had success with home-based programmes. Claire bought Kate a copy of *Let me hear your voice* – Catherine Maurice's personal account. Both her children are autistic and are now in mainstream education.

Kate and Michael were inspired.

But they didn't make much progress. Structure and consistency are integral to the Lovaas formula. It demands the creation of a structured environment that the autistic child can learn to understand. Kate and Michael live in chaos. Irregular hours. They'd clear a space whenever they had a moment to spare and launch into an activity quite unrelated to the day before. Or the day ahead.

They made zero progress with Amy. She seemed to have retrogressed each time we saw her.

Her parents were desperate. They decided they needed

professional help. They advertised for a teacher – put additional financial strain on their stretched resources. Their income had always been of a rather intermittent nature. We'd have been happy to contribute but we didn't know how to broach the subject. We sent a message via Claire's mother – and got a frosty decline. Kate didn't want Claire's help.

They employed a succession of teachers, none of whom had any qualifications in autistic education. A Masters student, busy on her thesis. A newly qualified college graduate who couldn't find a teaching post. A middle-aged social worker who'd been retrenched because of the government's transformation programme. All they had in common was the low salary they were prepared to accept. Plus their lack of specific training.

It wasn't a winning combination. Kate dismissed them, one by one. Too cold. Too impatient. Amy didn't seem to like them. The last one left of her own accord – she didn't like Amy. They were getting nowhere. They both looked dreadful. Kate was too thin, with dark hollows under her eyes. Amy never slept through the night. Michael looked exhausted – as if someone had switched his light off.

It became impossible to endure an afternoon with Amy.

I thought Claire had taken on more than she could handle.

*

As an actuary, Claire's familiar with statistical method. Her work is based on the principle of cause and effect. Actuarial models require a specified cause as a basis – it makes autism as difficult to deal with as astrology in terms of projected outcomes. There are so many possible variations that the equation becomes invalid.

I was much more interested than Claire in the reasons for Amy's inexplicable behaviour. I found a multitude of possibilities. Genetic influences. Identical twins, with a one hundred per cent overlap of genes, are more likely to suffer from autism than fraternal twins. Is an autism gene the culprit? A cluster of genes? Is it caused by a virus? A reaction to a childhood vaccination? Do toxins and pollutants make a contribution?

Claire says it's not important. Amy's autistic. That's a fact. It won't help to know why. But I'm curious . . .

If I was asked to summarise what's wrong with Amy, I'd say that she lacks the normal capacity for coherence. She never seems to see the bigger picture. She can't get the gist of a situation. It's as if she's lacking some central filter. At the end of a day, the rest of us decide what to remember and what to discard. I don't think Amy can do that. She can't forget unimportant detail so the main events are swamped.

There must be a rational explanation. I found Paul Shattock's case for autism as a metabolic disorder most persuasive, even though the medical jargon was unfamiliar. Elevated serotonin levels. Intense opioid activity. Disruption of the central nervous system. The advantages of a diet free of gluten and casein. Claire just shrugged her shoulders.

Her focus is on treating the effects. Medical opinion supports the idea that although autism can't be cured, it can be treated. Statistics don't favour one intervention above another but behaviour modification is the route she's

chosen. ABA. Applied Behaviour Analysis. *The Me Book* –
Ivor Lovaas' brainchild – has become a well-thumbed code
of reference on her bedside table. She opted for his
methods – not because she's sure they're going to work –
but because his approach seems tailor-made for her.

Lovaas' programme is highly structured. All activities
are broken down into manageable bites. It demands a high
degree of consistency from the teacher – and that comes
easily to Claire. She's even more organised than my mother.
Everything's in the same place and happens at the same
time. Order is a way of life for Claire.

Our home's an ideal environment for Amy.

The family room in our town house had always been a
bit of a misnomer. Apart from our lack of family, the décor
is stark. Minimalist furnishings. It doesn't encourage visitors
to make themselves comfortable and put their feet up on
the table. Anna's the only thing that ever changes places in
our house – and even she seldom moves out of her favourite
position. Claire converted the family room into a workroom from which she ran her Amy programme. One wall's
become a billboard. She pins up lists of the activities she
plans to cover every day. Detailed lists. Like tooth brushing.
Turn on the tap. Pick up the toothbrush by its handle. Wet
it. Turn off the water. Pick up the toothpaste, using your
other hand. Remove the cap. Put the cap down. Apply the
toothpaste to the brush. And so on.

I counted over twenty steps. Each one accompanied by
a verbal command. By visual prompts. By praise and
affirmatives. Provisions for time out on the days she won't
cooperate. Claire gradually fades the commands. She's
reached the stage where she only has to say 'Brush teeth',

for Amy to go through the entire routine unaided. It's a bit like Pavlov's dogs but at least she can do it. It's something.

Educating Amy is a slow, painstaking process. Claire sees her for as many as eight hours a day during the week. She keeps records of everything that happens. Or doesn't happen. That's another section on the billboard. Meticulous accounts. Date. Time. Frequency. Notes on each specific entry. I don't know how Claire tolerates the boredom. She says the process of habituation is less efficient in autistic people. Each time an experience is repeated, it appears as fresh and new so continued repetition of a particular activity isn't as mind-blowing as it would be to a normal person.

I believe Claire's also autistic so perhaps it's the same for her. It explains why she was so successful as an actuary.

She's also been successful as Amy's teacher, although it's not easy to measure the progress. Behaviour modification is based on small steps and the rewards are similar. Claire lights up at the smallest sign of breakthrough.

'I think I got somewhere today,' she told me one evening after Amy left. 'She seemed to be concentrating. She carried out all the tasks I set her. Looked me in the eye. Perhaps I'm getting somewhere at last.'

But the next day was different. Amy wouldn't cooperate at all. She gave no sign of recognition when Kate dropped her off that morning. It was as if it was the first time she'd ever seen Claire.

It takes stamina to persevere with an autistic child.

※

Claire didn't have to do it on her own. Amy's education

became a family mission. Claire's mother wasn't much use. She loved Amy unconditionally. She wasn't motivated to try to rewrite her granddaughter.

But help was available from an unexpected source. My mother proved invaluable. My marriage had left her with an empty nest of monumental proportions. I'd been her full-time focus for over forty years. Claire replaced her as my medical adviser. There was no further need to keep her records up to date. To comb the supermarket shelves in search of food that would both tempt my taste buds and keep my sugar levels on an even keel. Although we kept in constant contact, I have no real idea how she filled her days once she retired from the municipality.

Amy's problems were the answer to her prayers.

Autistic people are usually visual thinkers. Claire makes extensive use of picture cues. Visual descriptions of instructions. My mother became a specialist in illustrations. Neat cardboard squares. What she couldn't draw, she traced. She built up an extensive collection of children's colouring books. Claire's programme for Amy included regular outings. My mother drew pictures to show Amy what she could expect to find when she left the familiar walls of the workroom. Claire went through them all before departure. Handed her cards along the way, to remind her what was coming next. It was a system that worked well.

I went with them to Pretoria Zoo one Saturday morning. My mother drew up a zoo series. Amy putting on her shoes and hat. The car. The turnstile. Tickets. The cable car. Up and down. All the different animals. Even the final icecream. We all enjoyed ourselves. We looked just like a normal family. Granny and daddy with a pretty little girl between them. Mummy out in front, scouting around for potential hazards. Amy behaved beautifully. No one would have guessed she was autistic.

Not unless they saw the lion she drew on her return. We didn't show it to her mother.

It sounds as if we cut Kate and Michael out completely – but they remained central to Amy's education. Claire cast them both in specialist roles. They were the chief providers of positive reinforcement for Amy. We dealt with bread and butter issues – Kate and Michael made life fun for Amy. Kate was a wizard when it came to make-believe. Charades. She acted out stories and Amy had to find words to describe what she was doing. Her vocabulary was extended. The supermarket. The park. The circus . . .

Kate has so much imagination. I've watched her make a witch's brew with pots and pans and pumpkins. Amy had to drop the ingredients into the cauldron. Pick out the picture of a frog. A lizard. A bolt of lightning. She learned new nouns and verbs. To add. To mix. To pour. I could see she was making progress. It was good for Kate's morale to see that she was making as important a contribution as her sister. Claire bought a surgical brush. Amy learned to lie down on a blanket while her mother brushed her body gently. Up and down. Over and over. Claire said it helped reduce tactile defensiveness.

And maternal anxiety . . .

It was Michael who really made Amy come alive. Music therapy's particularly successful with autistic children because it's non-verbal. It was remarkable to watch Amy's response to her favourite songs on the piano. She'd clap and stamp her feet. She knew the words to Old MacDonald.

Raindrops Keep Falling On My Head. Kate cut holes in an old umbrella. Held it over Amy's head while she was dancing, slowly emptying a jug of water. Drops fell on Amy's upturned face as she danced below.

We were quite a team.

The only jarring note was Michael's mother. I know astrology's a science dating back to early Egypt. I shouldn't dismiss it as mumbo-jumbo but I've little confidence in theories that can't be statistically verified. I was sceptical the day she waxed on about the quartz singing bowl she's introduced into Amy's musical therapy.

'I bought it in Tibet,' she told me. 'It's made of a combination of three metals, mixed with pure quartz.' She circled the rim with a soft suede mallet. 'Listen to that,' she whispered. 'The sound's creating a sacred space for Amy. It balances the chakras. Helps you reach a tranquil place. It'll make her world quieter and more peaceful.'

I can't remember the rest of her lengthy explanation. I wasn't concentrating because I don't like her. I got the impression she was trying to impress her audience with her knowledge of ancient Eastern mysticism. I don't think she has any real interest in helping Amy. I also sense that she's negative towards Kate – ever since we heard Amy's diagnosis. I've spent much of my life on the alert for negative vibrations. My radar scans them out, even if they're not directed specifically at me.

Perhaps she influenced Michael. Turned him against Kate. There's a negative dimension in their relationship that was never there before.

A recent incident made me uneasy. Claire and I had been to the opening night of Kate's new show – a revival at the

Civic of Peter Nichols' savage, penetrating play. *A Day in the Death of Joe Egg*. It's billed as a comedy but we didn't find it funny. Perhaps the subject matter is too close to home. It's about a married couple with a severely retarded daughter. Kate plays the wife – she and her husband act out bizarre comic games with their afflicted daughter. I left the theatre, moved and shocked. I handed the review to Michael when he came to pick up Amy.

Joe Egg is a modern classic – funny, moving and intellectually stirring. Kate Templeton stands out in this performance as she fluctuates between defiant optimism at the smallest sign of progress and fitful despair. Her performance is made more poignant by the fact that she has a handicapped child herself. You can sense that she has first-hand knowledge of the sacrifices demanded. Her stubborn refusal to give up on her daughter, despite her limitations, is profoundly moving.

Michael scanned the words in silence. He crumpled up the paper and threw it on the floor.

*

Kate eventually changed her mind about the school for autistic children in Pretoria.

Claire continued her home-programme for two years. Step by step. Block by block. She was immersed in Amy's education. She'd have been willing to continue but Kate was stressed about her sister's shelved career – particularly as her own continued to flourish. She was also anxious about the need for social interaction with other children. Amy was making progress but Kate didn't think she'd cope in mainstream education. She was too solitary. The four of us – and our assorted mothers – were the only ones in Amy's life.

We all agreed that she should be eased into a classroom situation. Linda Fenton interviewed her again and agreed to accept her into the pre-school class at Unica.

It was the right decision because it made us stop feeling sorry for Amy. We saw how much worse it could have been. We knew that Amy was classified as high-functioning but we didn't have a real concept of what that meant until she started at Unica.

We were all excited when she was given a speaking part in the annual Christmas concert. She was cast as one of a group of moonbeams. The entire family knew her line, verbatim. *I am a silver moonbeam – I light up all the flowers in the garden when the sun goes out at night.* No line was ever more rehearsed. Bribery was standard practice – she could have started a chocolate factory with the rewards she received each time she said it. Michael played the moonbeam dance on the piano and she circled round on tiptoe, arms held high above her head.

The anticipation was tangible as we set out for Pretoria that morning. I took the morning off work. Claire and I collected her parents and my mother and we drove out to join Kate and Michael and the star of our show. Even our astrological connection made the effort. She looked as weird as ever as she joined us – we'd arrived half an hour early to ensure our front row seats.

It was one of those Pretoria mornings when the sky is impossibly blue – it's hard to beat a highveld summer. The stage was set up in the garden. The teachers had obviously gone to a huge amount of trouble. There was a canvas set, alive with trees and flowers. We applauded as they led their little charges through the routines they'd prepared.

We sat up to full attention as the piano struck up the familiar notes of the moonbeam melody. A troop of silver moonbeams tripped out from where they'd been waiting in the wings. They held hands and circled round the stage. Not in time to the music — but the audience wasn't critical. Amy was the most beautiful moonbeam. Frail and dainty in her silver dress which twinkled with sequins and strands of tinsel. Kate had made her a headband. Silver peaks of cardboard. Amy glued the glitter on herself.

We all had our cameras at the ready as our moonbeam stepped forward to say her line. We lit up like a line of glow-worms in our proud front-row seats. Amy was disconcerted by the sudden array of flashlights. Her face crumpled. She put out her hands to ward them off and stepped backwards. Curled defensively into a corner. Like a foetus, not prepared to leave the safety of the womb. Her teacher tried to coax her back but she wouldn't unfold. The moonbeam jingle finished and her fellow moonbeams left the stage.

It was a minor incident. Over in a moment. None of the other parents even noticed.

It seemed a cruel disappointment at the time.

Kate : Red. Multi-angled.

In retrospect, I recognise that my reaction to Amy's stage debut was ridiculous. Totally inappropriate. I behaved as if some ghastly catastrophe had taken place. I wept all the way home. Maybe that's why the gods decided I should have a child who's autistic. They thought my mood swings would be too much for a normal child to handle. It's lucky Amy can't read an emotional reaction. I would have made her feel so guilty. Over a single sentence.

I've got more insight into guilt than anyone. It's one emotion I'm glad my little girl will never feel.

Michael must also have been disappointed after all the rehearsals – but he didn't show it. He didn't show any sympathy for my reaction either. 'For Christ's sake Kate,' he snapped as I sniffed and snivelled in the seat beside him. 'Try to keep the matter in proportion. This wasn't opening night in a gala performance for the Queen of England. How can it possibly matter? You've had enough applause to melt the snow in an Arctic winter. You don't need another round for Amy. All she's missed is a bit of polite clapping from a handful of strangers at a morning tea. It certainly doesn't matter to her. Why does it matter so much to you?'

I know why it mattered.

From the moment I'd learned I was pregnant, I'd started writing a script for myself in this new and unexpected role. I planned to be more interesting than my mother. Less motherly. An inspiration. I'd anticipated a brand new audience. An adoring daughter. Hanging on every word I said, like I used to do with Michael's mother. She'd be surrounded by a gang of equally admiring friends – all clamouring to play at our house where Amy's amazing mother would act out the stories their own mothers merely read them. I knew Amy would stand out among them. She'd have her father's looks. His music and his sense of rhythm. She'd be as good on stage as I am. Even better. I expected to give birth to a chameleon – she'd change her colours according to the role that she was given. She'd shed her skin and become a new person on demand. Like me.

But those weren't the genes I gave her in the end. I know I'm wrong to feel cheated. I can't blame her for being Amy. She's completely helpless – she had to take what she was given. But in my heart, in my secret places, I'm bitterly disappointed that my maternal role's so different from the one I'd pictured.

Too big a part for me to handle . . .

✳

Amy has given me a new respect for mothers. Even if their children aren't autistic. I don't think motherhood is easy. Every mother starts off with high expectations – both of herself and of her child. But things go awry when a child turns out to be himself. Different from what you planned. I'm amazed by the otherness of other people. I try to get inside someone else's skin whenever I get a new role to play. I try to become the person that I'm playing. It's disconcerting to see the world from a different angle. From another point of view.

I've tried to do that with all the mothers in my life. Because of Amy, my opinions have shifted from my girlhood viewpoint. I've reassessed them in the light of their varied reactions to my daughter. Just as I've reassessed myself.

My own mother has been the most consistent. Supportive. Loving. Non-judgemental. I love my mother. I wonder what motherhood was like from her point of view. She must have felt that a cuckoo had landed in her nest when she hatched her mutant children. My mother handled our strangeness better than I've handled Amy. She accepted both of us, just the complicated way we were. And that's how she treats Amy. I'm ashamed of how superior I used to feel, how boring I considered both my parents.

Claire and I are lucky.

And so is Tony. My opinion of his mother has undergone a revolution. A full circle. I'd given both her and her son a zero rating before I had Amy. A fussy, boring municipal clerk and her tedious, actuarial son. They didn't seem to merit my attention as I swanned around, preening in the spotlight. But I've now spent hours talking to Tony's Mom. She understands the Amy situation better than anyone I know because of Tony's diabetes. Her life's also fuelled by guilt. She told me how she felt when her husband died – that she could somehow have changed what happened.

She and I start lots of sentences alike. If only . . .

We have problem children in common. Children with a serious medical condition – but her reaction's been opposite to mine. Less selfish. She devoted her whole life to Tony's welfare. She's now determined to get Amy back into the mainstream. She's more accepting of her fate than I am. Tony's mother isn't someone I should overlook. She's someone I should aspire to.

I remember the conversation we had when Amy's diagnosis was confirmed. 'I know how you must be feeling, dear,' she said patting my arm. Nodding. 'It seems so unfair. That's just how I felt when they told me Tony was diabetic. I'd lost his father and now he was also sick I felt so angry that it could happen to me twice. It seemed like a personal vendetta against me. Why me, I thought. And then I read the statistics about diabetes. It's almost an epidemic. So many wives and mothers have to face it. It made me think – why not me? It has to happen to someone. Why not me?'

That's one of my lines from *Joe Egg*. My latest starring role. The critics raved about my performance. They suggested I'd made the role so credible because I have a handicapped child myself. But Amy's handicap is nothing like Joe Egg's. Joe's hideously handicapped. Mentally and physically. *A human parsnip*. Journalists always quote that line. Amy's not comparable to Joe. She could have been much more affected than she is. She could have been far lower down on the autistic spectrum.

Why do I find it so hard to come to terms with everything that Amy isn't? With everything she'll never know or feel? I wish I could be more like Tony's mother. Why can't I repeat her words? Why do they still stick in my throat? Why can't I say that line?

Why not me . . .

I'm no better than Amy at her concert. Hiding under my chair. Refusing to utter the one sentence that could lead me forward into the future.

✳

My attitude to Michael's mother is the one that's shifted most. Amy's given me new insight. Taught me the danger of first impressions, of judging by appearances. I wrote off Tony's mother when I registered her floral summer dresses, buttoned tightly to the neck. Her sensible shoes. Her essential ordinariness. But I'm not as quick to pass a judgement as I used to be. I've rethought my relationship with Amy's other granny – just as she's done with me. Neither of us has proved as good a prospect as we seemed in the early days of my relationship with the central man in both our lives.

I was dazzled by Michael's mother's doctorate in astrology. Until I met her, I dismissed astrology as nonsense – I thought a horoscope was a load of junk concocted by journalists during their coffee breaks. She explained that

that was probably true of mass-media horoscopes. They're invalid. You can't generalise about horoscopes, any more than you can about people with autism. A qualified astrologer doesn't go by months. She needs the exact time of birth. Even a single minute can alter your forecast for the future.

It's a pity Amy wasn't born earlier. Or later. Maybe everything would be different.

Michael's mother taught me to respect astrology. For millennia, it's provided a coherent system for interpreting the world. She captured my imagination with astrology's rich symbolic language. She spun me magic tales of myths and legends. Astrology in the Book of Revelation. Synchronicities. Events in the past that related to specific planetary alignments. How they predicted the future. It was a hell of a lot more interesting than my mother's report on the annual general meeting of the PTA.

I trusted Michael's mother's opinion. I expected her to offer an explanation for Amy.

She was inspired by the birth of her only grandchild. She drew a natal chart, based on the sky settings at the moment of her birth. She didn't pretend to know Amy's future. She stressed that her chart dealt only with potential. She mentioned the influence of the planet Saturn. The planet of boundaries. Limitations. Something about emotions and the rising moon. I can't remember exactly what she said and I won't ask. She hasn't accepted Amy like the other mothers in my life.

Michael's mother is more like me. We were supposed to be the enlightened ones. We were liberal. Colour-blind. We voted for the ANC. For adoption rights for same-sex couples. We were scornful of parents who freaked out to learn their sons were gay. Michael's mother and I knew all the answers.

Until Amy. Then the conservative mothers – and the conservative sister – showed their true colours. They came out on top. They showed us up. Although she's never said so, I know Amy's most liberated grandmother hasn't come to terms with her grandchild's deficiencies. She doesn't accept her in the same way that my parents do. I never feel she's proud of Amy. Not like Claire and Tony.

She blames me for Amy. My daughter's similarity to Claire is obvious. She can see that the faulty gene cluster originated in my side of the family tree. She's not as warm as she used to be when I was merely a successful actress. Before I became the mother of her grandchild – the one who'd delivered her perfect son with a less than perfect daughter.

Michael had been a showpiece child. Good-looking. Talented. Confident. He'd perform on cue for all her friends. He was precocious. He'd stay up late to entertain them. He was all she needed to confirm her offbeat theories on child-rearing. On life in general. Amy's not like her father so she doesn't suit his mother. She never offers to babysit. She doesn't drop in. She used to have us round to drinks with all her arty friends. She liked to show us off – her perfect son and his semi-famous wife. Her granddaughter doesn't fit the bill.

She's ashamed of Amy.

I tell myself it doesn't matter. I hate Michael's mother. And all her fucking friends. That's an adjective I use often. I can see my mother wince as I drop it into every second sentence that I utter. It used to be a verb. A private, drenched-in-pleasure verb. It related only to us. To me and Michael. But it's been downgraded to an adjective today.

Amy's changed even my parts of speech.

I've applied that adjective to her. Fucking Amy. That's what I think when she messes up my plans. I mutter it in private. In my secret places where I have to recognise that I'm like Michael's mother. That I sometimes see my child as an obstacle to the route I've mapped out for my life.

I shock myself.

I knew I was a fraud when I stepped out to a standing ovation on the opening night of *Joe Egg*. I'd portrayed a mother who'd sacrificed everything to support a hopeless case. Her job. Her marriage. All her dreams. My performance was convincing. Everyone could feel the way I'd suffered. It's a great play – but it's not a reflection of my private trauma with my autistic daughter.

The critics were wrong about that.

All the mothers in my life must have made mistakes – it's part of the human condition. Even Mother Teresa knelt down before the priest and made confession. But none of them are in my class. I give a new dimension to the concept of motherhood.

I still can't believe I did it. I'm the worst mother on the planet.

✳

Michael was away the night before it happened – he had a function at Eagle's Nest in the Magaliesberg and they told him they'd give him a room if he'd continue playing after midnight. I'd started rehearsals for *The Syringa Tree* – David had struggled to get the rights and I'd been to three auditions before I got the part. It's an amazing play – about a child growing up in the height of the apartheid era. Maids and madams. I wanted that part more than I ever wanted anything before.

I'd had a close relationship with our family maid when I was growing up. Agnes is dead now but to me, she was more a part of our family than Claire. She was always old, even when I was a child. She worked for my grandmother all her life. When they moved into their retirement village, Agnes moved in with us. Into the servants' quarters, naturally. She was part of the family but she didn't eat or sleep or bath with us. No one ever asked why. South Africa's still a complicated country, despite the progress we've made. Agnes looked after Claire and me when my mother was at work. She watched me rehearse my roles at school. She laughed and waved her hands and clapped, slipping in and out of Xhosa. The relationship I had with Agnes was central to my childhood. I got the part because of her.

I've never met the writer though my mother and I saw her perform the play in New York. Pamela Gien. She's an ex-South African – I hate that term. No one is ever called an ex-American when they emigrate. I'll always say I'm South African, no matter where I end up living. You have to be South African to play this role. You need a South African bloodstream to know what it's about – the mud, the syringa berries, the nanny, the emigration. Leaving Africa. A glass wall at the airport, barricading the past and the future. It's exhausting to watch, let alone to play. Pamela Gien's astonishing. She spoke for at least a hundred minutes.

All alone. Twenty-four characters to coordinate with sound and lighting cues. Accents, physicalities, ages, sexes. It's a role that challenges every aspect of your being – as an actor, as a woman, as a South African.

I've got the cutting from the New York Times where Pamela Gien talks about the role. She said she monitored the things she ate. No dairy – it causes mucus. No smoky environments. No long conversations – to conserve her voice for the ordeal that faced her every night. She said she had no social life at all while she was performing *The Syringa Tree*.

I had no social life either. But I did have Amy . . .

She didn't sleep at all that night. The seventeenth of November. I'd picked her up from my mother's after a six-hour rehearsal. It's a daunting part, drenched in guilt and shame. I didn't know it well enough. I had to spend time on it. I had to absorb every line into my psyche.

I had to be alone.

But Amy wouldn't go to bed. She wouldn't stop running. She ran up and down the passage. Over and over. On wooden floors. It sounded like thunder. It drove me insane. I put down the script and went into the passage. I stopped her in midflight. Picked her up and held her.

'It's sleep time darling,' I told her. 'Time for sleeping.'

She was rigid in my arms. It was like holding a bar of iron. And then she started screaming. And screaming. And screaming. I was desperate. I put her in her bedroom and closed the door behind me. I went back into our bedroom. I pulled the cover over my head but I could still hear her screaming. A rising crescendo. And then she started hammering on the door . . .

I opened it and let her out into the passage. Eventually. She started running again. Backwards and forwards, from one end to the other. But she did stop screaming so the thundering floorboards felt almost like a breakthrough. I sat on my bed, legs crossed, script open. I tried to focus but the words swam and danced across the page. A blur of black and white. A light was flashing in my head. Jumbled words. They made no sense at all.

When she fell asleep there were just two hours left till morning. I didn't dare move her from the corner where she'd crumpled. I tiptoed to her with a blanket but I was scared. Amy doesn't like certain textures. Sometimes. You never know how she'll react. I was too frightened to touch her. It was chilly for November so it was hard to inch my way back into my bedroom with the blanket. My warm bed. Her cold corridor. It was impossible to fall asleep – in spite of my exhaustion.

I must have dozed. The light woke me. Amy was standing in my bedroom doorway. On tiptoe. She could reach the switch. She flicked it on. And off. And on again. I felt a scream rising in my throat. Bile, with words imbedded.

Stop it. Stop. Stop.

I forced myself to focus. I saw my child, delicate with tangled hair. A thin crumpled nightdress – too thin for the unexpected cool of the November evening. I got out of bed and crossed the floor. I held out my arms and felt the smallness of her body as she curled into me. I turned out the light and we lay together, united by exhaustion. Warm under the duvet. Mother and child. I could feel her cold limbs warming as we fell asleep.

But morning came. The fucking sun came up and forced

an entry through the curtains. Brazen. Bright. Bloody awful. I grumbled up and showered, my thoughts as crumpled as the un-ironed shirt I hauled out of the basket on the kitchen floor. I opened the fridge. It didn't look much like Bill Cosby's. His children always seem to find a pile of chicken drumsticks and a cold buffet. I unearthed some ancient yoghurt and a glass of juice. Amy poured both on the floor.

She's also tired I told myself, as I mopped the floor through gritted teeth.

It was easier for Michael to pick Amy up from my mother's so I said I'd meet him there. My rehearsal was only at eleven o'clock so I'd have time to get to Pick 'n Pay. Larry and Elaine were coming for a quick supper before they left for Cape Town and there was no fucking food. Fuck was the only word that came to mind as I did a mental survey of the day that stretched ahead. Especially when I picked up my script from beside the bed where it had fallen in the early hours of the morning. It might as well have been written in Chinese. I felt a knot of panic when I thought how David would react when I started stumbling.

I never took Amy to Pick 'n Pay. She had an allergy to supermarkets. The lights. The shelves. The people. The fucking carols. It was nearly December. Jingle Bells and Christmas cheer were company policy at Pick 'n Pay. Santa was at the entrance ringing a jovial bell when we arrived. Amy went into immediate hysterics. I knew she'd bite him if I let him advance any further. I flung her in a trolley and charged down the aisles at a speed that would have left Michael Schumacher breathless. I threw in random tins and bottles. Larry and Elaine weren't fussy.

I tried to bribe Amy with Smarties when we got to the

queue at the till.

There was a short silence while she gave the box her full attention. She opened the flap and looked intently at the orange disc in her fingers. I held my breath as she put it in her mouth. There were only two trolleys ahead of us. Not very full trolleys – not those trolleys that would feed a normal family for decades. It shouldn't take long . . .

Amy spat out the Smartie. She started to cry. She turned the box of Smarties upside down. A box of Smarties scatters far and wide if you turn it upside down at trolley height. My hands were shaking as I scrambled on the floor. Aware of public judgement. Aware of someone else's child in the trolley in front of me.

Just sitting there. Not screaming. Not spilling.

Normal.

I still had half an hour to spare when I got to my mother's. No one was home but I thought I'd try my script again. I grabbed a rug and Amy's bag of coloured blocks. She liked colours. I sat her on the lawn beside the pool. She sometimes liked to put her hand into the water. To splash her fingers. Like a real child. I turned my attention to the blocks. I piled them into a multicoloured pyramid. Maybe she'd like to knock them over. Or throw them at the dog. Maybe she'd like to do something while I looked at my script . . .

'Look Amy,' I started, turning round from my construction.

She had my script in her hand. She was scribbling on the pages in a dark thick koki pen. Scrubbing round and round in circles. Whorls of blue across the words. I heard the page rip. I wrenched the pen out of her hand. I heard myself screaming.

'No! No! No! Don't do that!'

I took her by the shoulders and I shook her. I hit her. Over and over. Harder and harder. As she started screaming, I heard the phone ring in the house.

It stopped me.

I heard it ring and ring. I heard Amy screaming in rage. And in pain. I'd hit her hard. With all my strength. I saw the pool. She can't swim. She can't be left without supervision. Especially beside a pool. But I got up and went inside to answer the phone. It stopped ringing as I reached the table in the entrance hall.

And Amy stopped screaming.

I registered the sudden silence but I couldn't move. My limbs were turned to stone. Dread flowed through my veins. Tightened in a vice around my stomach. I was aware of the beating of my heart. I don't know how much time had passed until I heard Michael's key turn in the lock. He thought I'd had bad news. I was standing right beside the phone.

'Jesus Kate,' he said, catching me by the shoulders. 'You look awful. Who phoned? What's happened? Is it your mother?'

I had to force myself to answer.

'It's Amy.' I heard my strangled whisper. 'She was scribbling on my script. So when the phone rang, I left her by the pool.'

I'll never forget how Michael looked when he registered the words that I was saying. Disbelief. Horror. I stumbled when he pushed me out of the way and ran out into the garden.

I couldn't follow.

I couldn't face the implications of that silence.

✳

Murder. Culpable homicide. An accident?

Emotional terms. Loaded with guilt and judgement. Especially if they apply to you. I've given them a lot of thought since that November morning – what they have in common. How they differ. If you watch LA Law, you'll know it's linked to motive. The focus is on the victim. Was the target random or specific?

I curl away in horror when I recall my victim. I'm like a centipede, turning in upon myself. I can't confront my action. I can't look it in the eye. A child victim is the worst. Any child. Because children are vulnerable. And innocent. It's a risk to go on stage when a child's in the cast – she always steals the show. Any actor knows that. Imagine when the child concerned is yours. Not just a random child.

My little daughter.

I remember Amy on arrival. Blood-smeared. A wrinkled, ancient face. Tiny grasping fists. The love-tug at my breast. The curve of her cheek as she lay sleeping. And especially her eyelashes, dark and dreaming in her pillow. Everyone remarked on Amy's eyelashes. And her eyes – too large for so small a face. My delicate Amy. My frail princess, growing up with slender limbs and streaming hair. Translucent almost. An underwater child, evolving on a different planet . . .

How could I have chosen Amy as the target for my rage?

You'll find assorted victims if you download murder on the net. Sometimes the victim is the sinner – someone who got her just deserts. A bully, maybe. Abusive and threatening. A manipulator. The jury can be very understanding in a case like that. Or even in a love-crime. White breasts. Red lips. Open thighs. A judge has insight into jealous torment. Compassion can suspend a sentence in matters of the heart.

But there can be no forgiveness if the victim is a child – from neither judge nor jury. Especially a damaged child. They're the most helpless of all. Particularly if the accused is her mother. Mother and murder are both loaded concepts. They should be diametrically opposed. A mother gives life and nurtures. Love should be an active verb. Murder can never be a synonym for mother.

No judge could forgive a mother like me.

But I'm not in jail. I was never convicted of my crime. I've never had to face the consequence of what I did on the eighteenth of November. Because Amy didn't fall in the pool. She's autistic. An autistic child's attention is caught, rather than directed. If something catches Amy's eye, she shifts her focus straight away. She's instantly absorbed. No normal child her age can focus on a single topic for so long.

She was still on the rug where I'd left her at the pool edge – the deep-blue edge of danger. Certain death if she'd gone exploring. But Amy was staring up into the tree above her head. The neighbour's cat. Amy likes cats. It was basking in the jacaranda tree that overhangs from their yard into ours. It was late November so it was in full flower. A mass of fragile blossom. Lavender. No leaves until the rain comes. The cat was lying on the branch, as motionless as only cats can be. Maybe its tail flicked slightly. Just for a moment. That's all it would have taken to catch Amy's attention. To divert her.

To save her life.

Michael carried her inside. I was still standing by the phone. I couldn't believe Amy was in his arms. My drowned child. *Those are pearls that were his eyes.* Ophelia. Tumbled thoughts as I reached out and took her in my arms.

I'm sorry. Sorry. Darling girl. I'm so sorry. Kisses. Tears. And terror – Amy must have felt she was being assaulted. Again. I'd hit her hard enough to leave a bruise.

Michael and I both flinched as we undressed her.

I wasn't judged for what I know was murder. I saw the pool. I heard the phone. I made my decision. That equation equals murder. I thought it would be better. For everyone. At least it would stop the screaming. I wanted quiet. I wanted to learn my words.

I deserve the judge's harshest sentence.

But it's not an eye for an eye. Not like in the Bible. There's no tit for tat in this millennium. The death penalty's illegal in our brave new world. In spite of this, I've paid for what I did. Even though it didn't happen. Crime and punishment – they're braided inextricably together, like Siamese twins who share a vital organ. Like love and marriage – you can't have one without the other. I sound like a darker version of Doris Day.

I remember that split second every morning. I'm guilty as I lie undercover, waiting for the sun to rise and tint the garden. Or just before I fall asleep. Each time my special girl wakes up, I remember how I tried to lose her.

I've never told anyone. I've sealed my secret in a capsule, like an oyster with a dark pearl hidden in its secret core.

But Michael knows. He was there. I remember his face before he went to help her. He recognised that I'd made a decision. I was standing by the phone. Conscious of the danger. Not helping . . .

I didn't lose my little girl that morning but I lost Michael. We've never discussed it but I know he can't forgive me for what I could have done. He didn't leave me. Maybe he stays because of Amy. Perhaps he doesn't trust me enough to go. Maybe he stays for old times' sake – a tribute to all we had together. I don't know why he stays.

But I know that everything is different now. I've blotted out our magic. I was the magician who made it disappear. As if I wore a pointed hat with occult skills and sleight of hand. One minute it was there, cast in solid concrete. But I waved my magic wand and pouf! It vanished.

Gone forever.

Claire : Ice-blue. Triangular.

When I dropped Amy at school that day, I didn't drive away immediately. I watched her as she walked across the court-yard. Someone waved and she turned towards a cluster of blue-clad girls. The group parted to absorb her. She looked just like one of them.

I could see how far Amy had come as I watched her walk across the St Agnes playground that day.

St Agnes is also a special school but it's not like Unica. It's mainstream education. The school psychologist mentioned it when Kate asked if Amy would cope else-where. Pretoria's a long drive from Jo'burg on a daily basis. It was a tiring day for a little girl. And for our lift scheme.

We looked at other schools. Highly rated private schools which specifically promote inclusion as part of the school programme. Tony would have paid the fees without a second thought. But the kids who go there look much like the cars that drop them off every morning. You can tell they come from a BMW environment. There's an air of confidence and competition, even in the playground. They're embryo yuppies. Some of the Grade Ones have cellphones.

I went to a school like that and I didn't fit in at all. Kate looked as if she understood when I put forward a case for St Agnes. She and I have come almost as far as Amy.

St Agnes is a tiny convent, tucked away in a Melville corner. It's a shabby Victorian building which opened as a school over sixty years ago. It continues to function in that time warp. The school has only two hundred pupils – mainly the daughters of old girls and missionaries and scholarship winners from the townships. They still call them pupils at St Agnes. They haven't heard that learner is the current term in the new South Africa. The Oxford defines a pupil as someone who is taught. I suppose learner is a more active word. With a pupil, the focus is on being taught – a receptacle rather than a catalyst. That's how it is at St Agnes. There's a million miles between the blackboard and the rows of desks. The boundaries between pupils and teachers never overlap like they do in more progressive schools.

There's a different ethos at St Agnes. The girls from other schools wear short, snappy tartan skirts – some don't wear a uniform at all. The newer schools are co-ed – gender equality is as topical as learner. Not much is topical at St Agnes. The uniform hasn't changed since the school was opened. Teal blue tunics and a navy sash. Straw bashers with a teal and navy band. Knee-high stockings. Black laced shoes. Amy knows exactly what she must put on every day.

Half the teachers at St Agnes are nuns. I thought nuns were extinct in the new millennium. Catholics see things clearly, especially if they're nuns. The rules don't change. Bells ring on time. Register. Chapel. Lessons. Break. More lessons. Home-time. There are no surprises at St Agnes. Amy has the same teacher for everything – Sister Mary. Her voice is gentle as she tells the tales she's been telling since she started teaching. The pattern never changes.

It's perfect for Amy.

I'm not pretending a miracle's occurred. Amy wasn't the ringleader in the group I was watching. She hasn't turned into a clone of her mother. She's listening to a little blonde who's holding forth with much vivacity. But she is listening. She looks normal. Almost normal. Not odd enough for anyone to notice. She doesn't rock and scream. She's lost that vacant stare. She looks at me directly. Usually. Not always.

We've come a long way.

The psychologist warned Kate that it wasn't over. It would never be over. The wheels could fall off at high school when her teachers change every time the bell rings. The world that's waiting for Amy won't be like St Agnes.

I thought again of my old kaleidoscope as I sat watching Amy and her group of classmates. Blue dresses. A tree, decked out in the bright green leaves of spring. Nursery rhyme clouds. A red brick wall. The colours and shapes slotted in like they had in my kaleidoscope, all those years ago. All the pieces fitted like a jigsaw in that frozen moment.

I know the picture will change when I turn the dial. There'll be a blur of motion as the pieces realign themselves in new positions. Nothing in a kaleidoscope stays constant. There's no certainty about Amy's future. Even as I watch, the movements start. The bell rings and they amble off towards the classroom. They all look the same from the back. A squad of blue. I couldn't even tell which one she was.

But I'm not certain that we've led her forward, despite the words we've taught her. Despite the coping skills she's mastered. Amy doesn't draw any more. No more cats. Her sinuous, feline miracles are over. She's lost her magic flair. She's ordinary now.

Was it a fair exchange?

I'll never be completely sure.

Acknowledgements

While researching *Kaleidoscope*, I have drawn on the expertise of the authors listed in the bibliography, as well as articles posted on the Internet. In particular, I have relied on the work of Dr Uta Frith who introduced me to characters in literature exhibiting autistic traits, Darold A Treffert for his insights into autistic savants and Time-Life Books for their wonderful photographs on the birth process. The reviews of the plays mentioned in the text were adapted from articles posted on the Internet – many thanks to the writers concerned.

Through the organisation Autism, South Africa, I was introduced to doctors, teachers and parents of children with autism. I was constantly amazed at the amount of time these people were prepared to spend talking to me – I would have been unable to write this book without their insights and I acknowledge the contribution of each with sincere thanks.

The following people were particularly helpful:

My daughter Nicola who's always the first to read everything I write – and who always thinks someone will publish it.

Vicky Canning of the Sandton Literary Agency, for her meticulous and perceptive editing.

Jane Ranger, Pam Thornley and Claire Heckrath of

Penguin Books for all their hard work and good advice.

Jill Stacey and Jeanetta Moreton of Autism, South Africa.

Dr Cobie Lombard of Unica School for Learners with Autism.

Dr Lynn Holford of Transvaal Memorial Institute for Child Health and Development.

The staff, parents and children of the Key School for Children with Autism during 2001 – especially Maggie and Thomas Ziehl, Annie and Thairu.

Don Tubesing for his wise advice and help in promoting the book.

Elaine McLachlan for her encouragement and wonderful artistic ideas.

Bianca Amato, Philippa Dissel, Felicity Jackson, Lesley McIntyre, Karen Milner and Jill Worth for their help with background information and early readings.

And not forgetting The Girls who sat supportively under my feet at the computer for every word I typed.

Copyright credits:

The excerpt on page 14 is from *The Vagina Monologues* by Eve Ensler, published in 2001 by Random House, Inc, Villard Books 1745 Broadway, New York, NY 10019, and is reproduced by kind permission of the publishers. The extract from *Tommy* (page 139) is reproduced with the permission of Hal Leonard Corporation and BMG Music Publishing International.

Every effort has been made to trace copyright holders or their assigns, and the author and publishers apologise for any inadvertent infringement of copyright.

Bibliography

Frith, Uta. *Autism – Explaining the Enigma*. Blackwell Publishers. Oxford. 1989.

Grandin, Temple. *Thinking in Pictures*. Doubleday. New York. 1995.

Jordan, Rita. Assorted papers. Pretoria symposium on Autistic Spectrum Disorders. University of Pretoria. 2000.

Kustow, Michael. *Theatre@Risk*. Methuen Publishing Ltd. 2000.

Lovaas, Ivor. *The Me Book*. Prentice Hall. 1974.

LeDoux, Joseph. *The Emotional Brain*. Weidenfeld and Nicolson. London. 1998.

Lombard, JC. *Asperger's Disorder*. Unica School for autistic children. Pretoria. 2000.

Maurice, Catherine. *Let me hear your voice*. Robert Hale Ltd. London. 1994.

Shattock Paul, Whitely Paul, Savery Dawn. *Autism as a metabolic Disorder and Guidelines for Dietary Intervention*. University of Sunderland. 2000.

Treffert, Darold A. *Extraordinary People. An Explanation of the Savant Syndrome*. Bantam Press. London. 1989.

Williams, Donna. *Nobody, nowhere*. Doubleday. London. 1992.

Autism, South Africa. Assorted pamphlets for parents, doctors and teachers.